# Essential ENT Practice

# Essential ENT Practice

## A CLINICAL TEXT

### Rogan J Corbridge *BSc FRCS*

*ENT Specialist Registrar, Radcliffe Infirmary, Oxford, UK*

WITH CONTRIBUTIONS FROM

### William PL Hellier *FRCS*

*ENT Specialist Registrar, St George's Hospital, London, UK*

**ARNOLD**

A member of the Hodder Headline Group
LONDON • SYDNEY • AUCKLAND
Co-published in the USA by Oxford University Press, Inc., New York

First published in Great Britain 1998 by
Arnold, a member of the Hodder Headline group,
338 Euston Road, London NW1 3BH

Co-published in the United States of America by
Oxford University Press, Inc.,
198 Madison Avenue, New York, NY10016
Oxford is a registered trademark of Oxford University Press

Whilst the advice and information in this book is believed to be true and
accurate at the date of going to press, neither the author nor the publisher
can accept any legal responsibility or liability for any errors or omissions that
may be made. In particular (but without limiting the generality of the preceding disclaimer) every effort has been made to check drug dosages; however it is still possible that errors have been missed. Furthermore, dosage
schedules are constantly being revised and new side-effects recognized. For
these reasons the reader is strongly urged to consult the drug companies'
printed instructions before administering any of the drugs recommended in
this book.

*British Library Cataloguing in Publication Data*
A catalogue record for this book is available from the British Library

*Library of Congress Cataloging-in-Publication Data*
A catalog record for this book is available from the Library of Congress

ISBN 0 340 67704 X

Publisher: Fiona Goodgame
Production Editor: James Rabson
Production Controller: Sarah Kett
Illustrator: Peter Cox
Cover designer: Mouse Mat Design

Typeset in 9/12pt Frutiger by Scribe Design, Gillingham, Kent, UK
Colour reproduction by Tenon and Polert Colour Scanning Ltd, Hong Kong
Printed and bound in Great Britain by Cambus Litho Ltd, East Kilbride

# Contents

Introduction     vii

1    The ENT history and examination     1

2    Understanding investigations in ENT     11

3    The mouth, tonsils and adenoids     17

4    The salivary glands     31

5    The larynx     39

6    The oesophagus and dysphagia     61

7    The thyroid gland     71

8    The neck     79

9    The ear     89

10    The nose and nasopharynx     121

11    The paranasal sinuses     139

12    The ENT manifestations of AIDS and HIV infection     151

13    Procedures in ENT     155

14    Pharmacology in ENT     163

15    Glossary of common terms in ENT practice     167

Index     171

# Acknowledgements

I would like to thank all my teachers over the years, both in London and in Oxford without whose dedication and enthusiasm this book would not have been written.

I dedicate this book to my long-suffering and patient wife, Luisa, and our children Olivia, Alexandra and Max.

# Introduction

This book offers a modern and updated guide to ENT practice. It differs from most other text books covering this area of medicine, in that it is written not by eminent professors who were medical students a generation ago, but by trainees in ENT who remember only too well medical school days and therefore can recall what it was that we found difficult and why we were frustrated by the texts of the day.

The book is aimed primarily at medical students but we hope that general practitioners and those embarking in a career in ENT will also find this a useful and solid grounding in all aspects of the speciality.

Where at all possible we have tried to approach the subject in a problem orientated way, which we feel is far more relevant to the day-to-day practice of medicine, and also will help the student to prepare for battle with the examiners, where they will be faced with real patients with real problems.

Most chapters have an 'Overview' of the diseases which affect the region under discussion. It is not intended that the student should try to memorize these rather daunting lists, but rather that he/she will use them to gain an appreciation of the diversity of conditions which may affect the ear, nose and throat. In each overview, the student will be able to identify the more common conditions since these are presented in bold. Also, we hope that since the lists are organized in a structured way (following the time honoured surgical sieve, so much beloved by the examiners) the reader will be able to use this to their advantage when revising or in a discussion. The more important or common conditions are selected from the overview for further discussion in the rest of each chapter.

Finally, the chapter on procedures in ENT aims to give a practical guide to general practitioners and casualty staff on the management of the more common emergencies which are frequently seen.

# 1

# The ENT history and examination

The history  2

Equipment required  4

Examination of the ear  5

Examination of the mouth, larynx and neck  8

Examination of the nose  10

# THE HISTORY

The history in ENT, as with all other branches of medicine and surgery, is of the upmost importance. The information gleaned during this part of the consultation will guide one towards particular areas during the examination and indicate which investigations may be appropriate; obviously this is essential if the doctor is to come to the correct diagnosis. The interactions during history taking form the foundation of a strong doctor – patient relationship. This is vital if any effective treatment plan, offered by the doctor, is to be acted upon by the patient.

## Structure of the history

The structure of the history is similar to medical school teaching across the world.

### The history of the presenting complaint

This will include details of the main symptoms, their exact nature and duration, as well as any other associated or predisposing factors. Specific questions related to the system or systems in question should also be asked at this point. In general, unilateral symptoms should raise the level of suspicion since most conditions which have serious consequences such as tumours and malignancies are unilateral, at least initially.

### The past medical history

Previous or concurrent medical conditions which are relevant to the current problem, or those that may affect the patient's treatment or fitness for anaesthesia, must be determined and noted appropriately.

### The drug history

The doctor must enquire about drugs which may be directly relevant to the present ENT complaint, e.g. anticoagulants in a patient with a nose bleed or the use of aminoglycosides in patients with hearing loss. Also he/she should determine if the patient takes any other regular medication, prescribed or otherwise. A history of adverse drug reactions and allergies should also be taken.

### The social history

Here, details of the patient's employment should be noted. In some cases, details of their home environment may also be relevant. Alcohol intake and smoking history should also be determined.

## The nose

Many patients will complain of nasal obstruction; here, try to determine if this is uni- or bilateral. Is it constant or intermittent? Are there associated features such as sneezing, nasal itch or hayfever? If the patient complains of rhinorrhoea or postnasal drip, what is its quality? Features which may indicate sinus involvement in nasal pathology are pressure or pain in the cheeks, forehead or across the bridge of the nose; this is often associated with a 'muzzy head'. Unilateral epistaxis or blood-stained nasal discharge, nasal obstruction and facial pain or swelling must be recognized as the common presenting features of nasal tumours. One should enquire concerning defects in the sense of smell, i.e. loss of smell (anosmia) or unpleasant odours (cachosmia).

## The ear

Hearing loss is the commonest presenting complaint in diseases of the ear. Once again, a unilateral loss should raise the level of suspicion. Any history of previous noise exposure or family history of hearing problems may be relevant. In children with hearing problems, one should enquire about other congenital conditions and a history of birth or neonatal trauma and anoxia, as well as other serious childhood infections such as meningitis.

Pain in the ear (otalgia) and/or discharge from the ear (otorrhoea) are also common symptoms as is itch in the ears. The nature of any discharge from the ears should be determined. For example, is it simple wax, purulent, blood-stained or watery? Each of these may suggest a differing pathology. Foul-smelling otorrhoea is characteristic of cholesteatoma. Patients often complain of noises in the ears (tinnitus) and will often go into long and detailed descriptions of what they hear. Much of this is unhelpful in making the diagnosis. It is, however, important to recognize pulsatile tinnitus which occurs with serious vascular tumours or malformations. Popping and cracking noises in the ears are suggestive of eustachian tube dysfunction, as is a feeling of pressure within the ear.

Dizziness is another frequently encountered complaint. Here it is important to take a detailed history of its exact nature, any predisposing factors, associated symptoms and a general medical history. If after taking the history you do not have a suspected diagnosis, the examination and investigations are unlikely to give it to you!

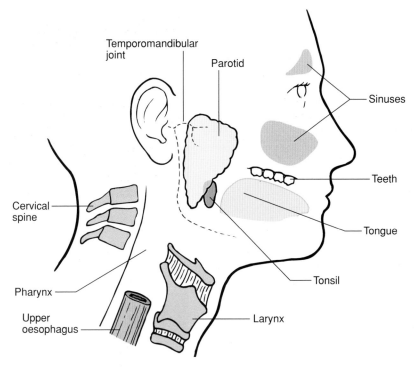

FIGURE 1.1 Causes of referred otalgia.

The facial nerve and chorda tympani are intimate relations of the ear and as a result, pathology may involve these structures and lead to an alteration in the sense of taste or facial weakness. These are symptoms which must be enquired about directly since the patient, not unreasonably, may fail to connect them with the ear, and therefore may fail to volunteer this vital information.

Pain in the ear (otalgia) may be due to ear problems which are usually evident on examination. However, the ear is also a common site for referred pain from many other sites within the head and neck, due to their shared innervation (branches of the same nerve supply different structures and hence irritation in one area may be perceived as pain in another), e.g. sinuses and teeth, temporomandibular joint, cervical spine, oropharynx and throat (Figure 1.1).

## The throat

When taking a history from a patient who complains of a hoarse voice, it is important to determine the duration and circumstances which preceded this symptom. For example, did it occur following a common upper respiratory tract infection, or as a result of shouting at a football match or (more worryingly) a gradual onset in a smoker? The professional history is important since it will determine if the patient is a professional or amateur voice user. Smoking and alcohol intake are also important facts to document.

Other common symptoms are a feeling of a lump in the throat, mucus in the throat and discomfort. Often these symptoms are features of innocent pathology. However, they may also be the presenting features of neoplasia. Acid reflux may also contribute to, or cause, throat problems and therefore other features suggestive of this must also be sought.

## The mouth and neck

Sore throat and tonsillitis along with intra-oral lesions such as ulcers on the tongue are the commonest conditions of the mouth seen in ENT practice. It is important to ascertain a good general medical history since a wide variety of systemic conditions such as anaemia and HIV infection can present with oral manifestations. In the case of swellings within the mouth, an increase in size or pain with eating is suggestive of salivary gland disease.

Patients with lumps in the neck *must* be referred to an ENT specialist, since only he or she has the equipment and expertise adequately to examine the likely primary sites from which secondary neoplastic neck node deposits may originate. When taking a history from such a patient, one must enquire about any symptoms from the likely primary sites such as the tongue, mouth, nose and throat.

---

**KEY POINTS**
**Neck Lumps**

All neck lumps must be referred to ENT since, if malignant, the primary site is likely to have arisen in the:

- Nasopharynx
- Oropharynx
- Tonsil
- Tongue base
- Pyriform fossa
- Larynx
- Upper oesophagus

---

A history of a preceding infection is suggestive of a 'reactive' node. Symptoms of weight loss, night sweats and malaise may suggest a systemic disease such as lymphoma or AIDS. Features of thyroid over- or under-activity should also be sought.

---

**KEY POINTS**
**Danger Signs in ENT History**

- Hoarse voice for more than 3 weeks (tumour)
- Foul-smelling otorrhoea (cholesteatoma)
- Unilateral foul nasal discharge in a child (foreign body)
- Unilateral nasal polyp/blood-stained rhinorrhoea (tumour)
- Unilateral deafness (tumour)
- Persistent lump in the throat (tumour)

---

# EQUIPMENT REQUIRED

Figure 1.2 shows the equipment which is commonly used in ENT practice.

## The head mirror

Good illumination is essential when examining all areas in ENT. The most commonly available and traditional method is using the head mirror. This has the advantage that it allows 'hands-free' illumination. Use of the head mirror is a valuable skill which is easy and quick to learn.

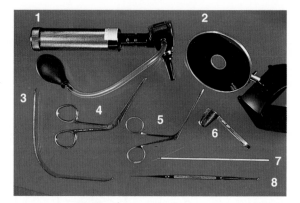

FIGURE 1.2 (1) Auroscope. (2) Head mirror. (3) Tongue depressor. (4) Tilley's nasal dressing forceps. (5) Crocodile forceps. (6) Thudicums nasal speculum. (7) Silver Nitrate cautery stick. (8) Jobson–Home probe.

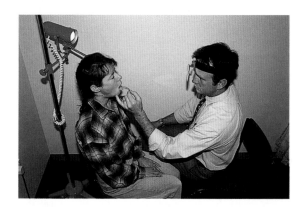

FIGURE 1.3 Using a head mirror. Note the positions of the light source, patient and examiner.

The basic principle of the head mirror is that light is reflected from the mirror onto the patient. The mirror is concave and thus the light is focused to a point. Also, it has a hole through which the examiner can look so allowing binocular vision. Correct positioning of the patient, the examiner and the light source is important (Figure 1.3).

## How to use a head mirror

Place the mirror over the right eye, close the left eye, and adjust the mirror so that you can look through the hole directly at the patient's nose. Now adjust the light and mirror until the maximum amount of light is reflected onto the patient. When the left eye is opened, you should have binocular vision and the reflected

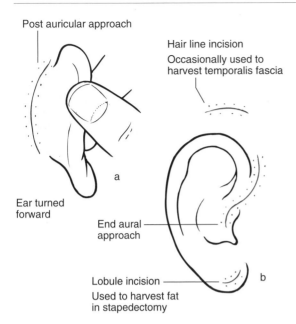

Post auricular approach

Hair line incision
Occasionally used to
harvest temporalis fascia

a

Ear turned
forward

End aural
approach

Lobule incision
Used to harvest fat
in stapedectomy

b

FIGURE 1.4 Surgical scars around the ear. (Look carefully –
they are often difficult to see.)

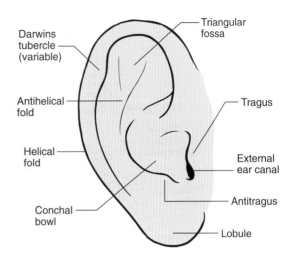

Darwins
tubercle
(variable)

Antihelical
fold

Helical
fold

Conchal
bowl

Triangular
fossa

Tragus

External
ear canal

Antitragus

Lobule

FIGURE 1.5 Nomenclature of the pinna.

light shining to the patient's nose. The focal length of
the mirror is approximately two feet. This means that
the reflected light will be brightest and sharpest when
examiner and patient are this distance apart.

# EXAMINATION OF THE EAR

## The external ear

The size, shape and position of the pinnae should be
observed. When examining the external ear, one
should also note the presence of surgical scars around
the ear (Figures 1.4 and 1.5). Also, the presence of
congenital abnormalities such as accessory auricles,
skin tags and pre-auricular sinuses should be noted.

## The auroscope

The auroscope should be held correctly in the left hand
when examining the left ear and the right hand when
examining the right ear. The external auditory meatus
(EAM or ear canal) should be straightened by gently
lifting the pinna upwards and backwards (Figure 1.6).
Choose the largest speculum that will comfortably fit
into the ear canal, since this will give the best view and
admit the most light. Then the auroscope is gently
inserted along the line of the ear canal. As with all
examinations, try to be methodical. Note, in turn, the
skin of the ear canal, the pars tensa with the handle

and lateral process of the malleus and the light reflex.
It is most important to pay particular attention to the
tiny strip at the top of the ear drum known as the pars
flaccida, since it is in this area that cholesteatomas are
first seen (Figures 1.7 and 1.8.) Some auroscopes have
a pneumatic bulb which can be attached. This allows
air to be puffed in and out of the ear canal, and with
experience the examiner can learn to assess the mobility of the drum.

## Tuning fork tests

These are simple tests used to assess patients' hearing
and are often extremely useful. However, it should be
appreciated that the pure tone audiogram is the gold
standard investigation.

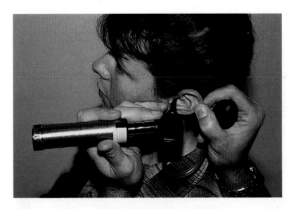

FIGURE 1.6 How to hold an auroscope. Note how the
auroscope is held in a 'pencil grip' and also how the little
finger rests on the patient's face. In this case, the pneumatic
bulb is also being used.

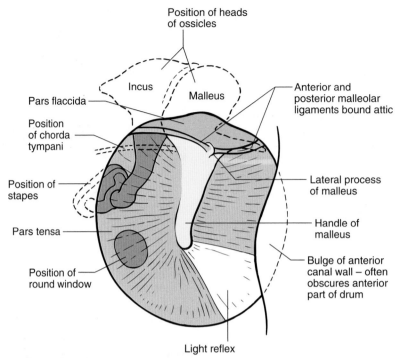

Position of heads
of ossicles

Incus

Malleus

Pars flaccida

Anterior and
posterior malleolar
ligaments bound attic

Position
of chorda
tympani

Position of
stapes

Lateral process
of malleus

Pars tensa

Handle of
malleus

Position of
round window

Bulge of anterior
canal wall – often
obscures anterior
part of drum

Light reflex

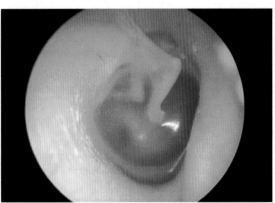

FIGURE 1.7 A normal right ear drum (otoscopic appearances).
Note: shaded structures are those which are sometimes seen
through a thin tympanic membrane or a tympanic
membrane perforation.

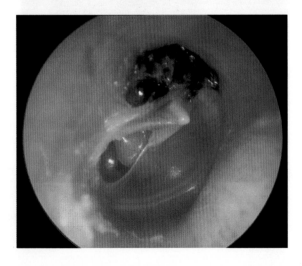

FIGURE 1.8 An attic cholesteatoma of the right ear. Note the
extension to the middle ear (the white mass seen through a
thin posterior segment of the ear drum). Reproduced with
the kind permission of Mr I. Botrill FRCS.

At first, tuning fork tests may seem complicated.
However, they are in fact quite simple and very useful.
Take a few minutes to read the following descriptions
and diagrams, in order to make sure you understand
them.

First, be sure that the tuning fork is the correct frequency for testing hearing, i.e. 512 Hz. The value of
these tests lies in determining whether the hearing loss
is a conductive type (i.e. some defect in the transmission of sound to the inner ear, for example a problem
with the ear canal, drum, middle ear and ossicles), or

sensorineural type (i.e. a defect either in the cochlea, auditory nerve or the central nervous system).

## Weber's test (Figure 1.9)

Here the tuning fork is struck and placed on the patient's forehead, nasal bridge or upper teeth (not if dentures are used!) and the patient is asked where the sound is best heard. The results can be summarized as follows:

- Unilateral or asymmetrical hearing loss
  Conductive type    localizes to the affected (worse hearing) ear
  Sensorineural type  localizes to the non-affected (better hearing) ear
- Bilateral or symmetrical loss of either type; the sound is heard equally in both ears

## Rinne's test (Figure 1.10)

This test determines how sound is best heard, through air or through bone (air conduction, AC; or bone conduction, BC). The tuning fork is held next to the ear for a few seconds; then it is placed behind the ear on the mastoid process. The patient is then asked which they can hear better. The results of this test can be summarized thus:

- Rinne positive (i.e. AC > BC): This is the response in normal ears, and in patients who have a sensorineural hearing loss in the test ear.
- Rinne negative (i.e. BC > AC): This is the response in a patient who suffers with a conductive hearing loss in the test ear.

The situation is complicated in one important situation, when the patient has a false-negative Rinne test. This occurs when the patient has a profound sensorineural hearing loss, or 'dead ear' in the test ear. In this situation, one would expect the Rinne test to be positive; however, a negative response occurs. This is explained by the fact that when testing hearing through air, nothing is heard in the test ear since it is 'dead'; however, when the tuning fork is placed on the skull, sound is transmitted through the skull base, not only to the 'dead' cochlea, but also to the normal cochlea on the opposite side where it is heard; therefore, the sound is perceived as louder via bone than air conduction (Rinne negative).

In order to counter this false result it is important that every time a negative response is achieved, the test is repeated. However, this time a masking noise is applied to the non-test ear using a Barany noise box; this has the effect of 'occupying' the cochlea on that side and thus a true positive response will be achieved.

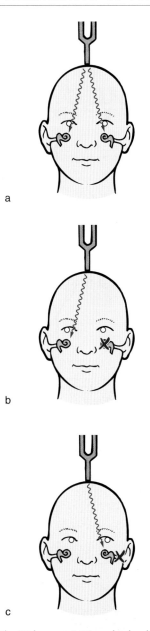

FIGURE 1.9 The Weber test. (a) Sound is localized centrally with equivalent hearing in both ears; (b) unilateral sensorineural deafness localizes sound to the better side; (c) unilateral conductive deafness localizes sound to the same side.

A simple way to apply masking is to rub the tragus of the pinna with your finger.

## Simple tests of hearing

The hearing can be tested in the clinic or surgery without any equipment at all. These tests are known as

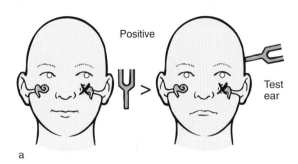

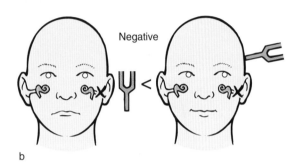

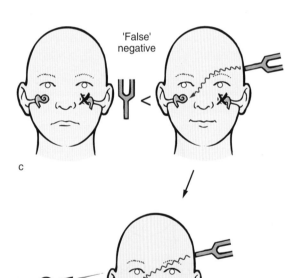

FIGURE 1.10 The Rinne's test. (a) Patients with normal hearing or a partial sensorineural deafness hear sound better through air than bone: a *positive* Rinne test; (b) conductive deafness leads to a *negative* Rinne test; (c) in profound deafness the test may also be *negative* but this false result may be detected by masking the good ear with a noise box.

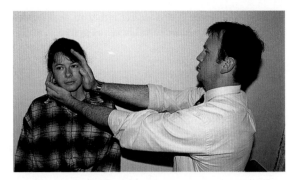

FIGURE 1.11 How to perform free field testing. Note the positions of the hands, one of which is shielding the patient's eye and the other is providing tragal rubbing. The test words are delivered at arm's length.

*whisper tests* or *free field tests* (Figure 1.11). The patient is asked to repeat a series of words or numbers which are given by the examiner at different volumes. Most people with normal hearing (hearing threshold 0–20 dB) should be able to hear a whisper delivered at arm's length. If the patient can only hear a normal conversational voice at the same distance, this would indicate there is a hearing threshold of approximately 30–40 dB. Loud conversational voice equates to approximately 40–60 dB and shouting 100–120 dB hearing thresholds. Once again the opposite ear should be masked using tragal rubbing and visual clues should be removed by shielding the patient's eyes.

# EXAMINATION OF THE MOUTH, LARYNX AND NECK

## The mouth

Examination of the mouth must be systematic and methodical. A good light is essential. Remember also to ask the patient to remove all dentures, since these may hide important pathology. Each of the following areas should be examined in turn. The tongue, looking first at its upper surface, then the edges and under surface. Pay particular attention to the side of the tongue right at the back; this is known as 'coffin corner' since carcinomas of the tongue may easily be missed in this region. Look at the floor of the mouth, the lower teeth and gum line, both on its inner and outer surfaces. Use a tongue depressor to lift the cheek away from the upper teeth and look at the parotid duct opening, opposite the upper second molar tooth. Now turn your attention to the upper teeth and gums, and from here

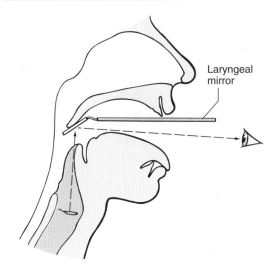

FIGURE 1.12 Indirect laryngoscopy.

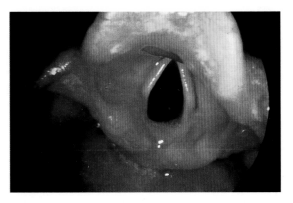

FIGURE 1.13 Nasendoscopic view of the larynx.

look at the hard and soft palates. Note the presence or absence of tonsillar tissue and the surface of the posterior pharyngeal wall. Test the movements of the tongue and also the palate by asking the patient to say 'Aahh'. Finally, place a gloved finger into the mouth and feel the base of the tongue and the floor of the mouth. Now a second hand placed under the jaw allows the submandibular gland to be palpated.

## The larynx

Much information can be gained simply by listening to the patient's voice. They may have a hoarse voice suggestive of a lesion on the vocal fold, or they may have the weak breathy voice, with a poor 'bovine' cough suggestive of a vocal fold palsy. However, in order to confirm the diagnosis, the larynx must be viewed. The traditional method is using the head mirror and an angled laryngeal mirror held at the back of the mouth, against the soft palate (Figure 1.12). Nowadays, fibre-optic endoscopes are generally preferred since they give a superior view and are tolerated by almost every patient (Figure 1.13).

## The neck

Once again, it is important to ensure that the examination is systematic and methodical in order to avoid missing a small, or second mass. Exactly which system is used does not matter as long as all regions are palpated. The following is a suggested method (Figure 1.14). Start at the mastoid tip, work forward to feel the post- and pre-auricular lymph nodes; from here, move

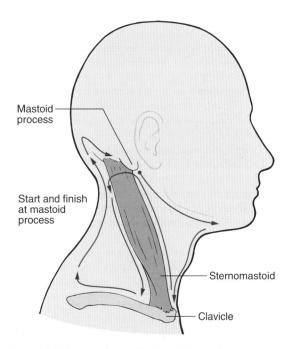

FIGURE 1.14 Systematic examination of the neck.

forward to feel the parotid followed by the submandibular region. The hands meet under the chin in the midline; now move down the midline, feeling in turn each lobe of the thyroid gland and the isthmus. From the suprasternal notch, follow up the anterior border of the sternomastoid muscle back to the mastoid tip once more. Now follow the posterior border of the sternomastoid muscle down to the clavicle; move laterally along the clavicle and to the anterior border of the trapezius muscle, palpating the posterior triangle as you go; follow right round to the midline posteriorly. Feel the cervical spine up to the skull base and note any occipital lymph nodes. Finally move forward along the skull base to finish once more at the mastoid tip.

# EXAMINATION OF THE NOSE

The shape of the nose and its size relative to the rest of the face, as well as any cosmetic deformity, should be noted. Next, the airway on each side of the nose should be tested. This can be done by occluding each nostril in turn and asking the patient to sniff in. At this point, also look for collapse of the soft tissues of the nose during inspiration, so-called *alar collapse*.

When occluding the nostril, this should be done by placing the thumb over the nasal aperture rather than pressing on the side of the nose. Another way to test the airway is to hold a cold shiny surface, such as a metal tongue depressor, under the nose and look for the pattern of misting that occurs as the patient breathes.

Next, the nasal tip should be elevated. This gives an opportunity to examine the nasal vestibule for any small lesions which may otherwise be covered up by the blades of a nasal speculum. Examination of the nasal cavity demands a good light source, for example a head mirror. A thudicums speculum is used to hold open the nasal aperture and then systematic examination of the nasal cavity can follow. If a head light and thudicums speculum are not available, an auroscope and ear speculum can be used instead. Each area of the nasal cavity should be examined, in turn looking at the septum, floor of the nose and then the lateral wall where the inferior and middle turbinates will often be seen (and are frequently confused with nasal polyps) (Figure 1.15).

One should note the appearance of the nasal mucosa, its colour, surface and hydration. Examination of the postnasal space requires special

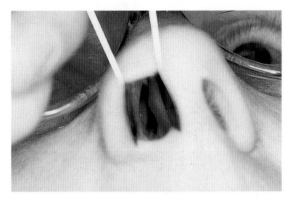

FIGURE 1.15 Note the anterior end of the middle turbinate which can be seen projecting from the side wall of the nasal cavity. This is often confused with a nasal polyp by the less experienced examiner.

equipment, either a small mirror introduced via the mouth, or a fibreoptic endoscope via the nose. It must be remembered that the ear and nose are connected by the eustachian tube, therefore nasal pathology may produce ear problems. Therefore, examination of the nose is incomplete without also examining the ears.

## KEY POINTS
### Principles of ENT Examination

- Good illumination
- Practise your technique
- Correct equipment
- Be methodical

# 2

# Understanding investigations in ENT

Investigations in otology 12

Investigations in rhinology 15

Allergy testing 16

This chapter is not intended to provide an exhaustive list of every investigation carried out in ENT practice. We will not, for example, discuss the details of the full blood count. Instead, we shall briefly discuss those important investigations which are performed largely, or entirely, within ENT practice as well as those which are unlikely to be encountered in other spheres of medicine.

# INVESTIGATIONS IN OTOLOGY (Table 2.1)

## Tests of hearing: audiometry

Simple tuning fork tests (Rinne's and Weber's tests) have been covered in Chapter 1. The hearing tests carried out in the ENT clinic are able to determine the degree of hearing impairment and also the type of hearing loss, i.e. conductive or sensorineural. Moreover, they can detect the relative contribution of each type in a mixed loss.

TABLE 2.1 Investigations in otology and rhinology

| INVESTIGATION | COMMON TESTS IN EVERYDAY USE | LESS COMMON BUT USEFUL INVESTIGATIONS |
|---|---|---|
| Otology | Tuning fork tests Pure tone audiogram Tympanometry Magnetic resonance imaging (MRI) | Speech audiogram Electrocochleography Brain stem evoked response Cortical evoked response Otoacoustic emissions Stapedial reflexes |
| Rhinology | Computed tomography (CT) sinuses Skin tests | Peak inspiratory nasal airflow Acoustic rhinometry Saccharin taste test Ciliary brushings Smell bottles Radio-allergo-absorbent test (RAST) |

Most tests rely on the patient indicating that they can hear a sound, these tests are therefore *subjective* and depend upon the patient's ability to understand what the test requires of them, and to perform the test to the best of their ability. In some patients, such as small children, or where there is some concern as to their honesty, other *objective* tests of hearing are required. Unfortunately, these tests are less accurate than properly performed subjective tests, and therefore are not used for routine hearing assessment.

In the past, when a patient was found to have a unilateral sensorineural hearing loss, a range of complex audiological tests were required in order to try to support or refute the diagnosis of an acoustic neuroma (a rare type of tumour affecting the VIIIth cranial nerve). This whole area of audiometry has now been largely superseded by scanning, in particular magnetic resonance imaging (MRI).

## Subjective tests of hearing

### The pure tone audiogram

This is the most commonly performed hearing test and is used to determine the patient's hearing 'threshold'. A series of tones are presented to the patient via headphones, first to one ear and then the other. The patient is asked to respond each time they hear the sound. The quietest sound that the patient can hear is documented and the whole process repeated for another frequency. The resulting audiogram is shown in (Figure 2.1). Tests of the 'normal' population show that 95% have air-conduction thresholds better than 25 dB over four frequencies. This level is taken as the lower limit of normal. Sounds can also be delivered to the patient via a bone-conducting vibrator placed onto the mastoid process. Thus, both air- and bone-conduction thresholds can be determined. In order to achieve accurate results, the non-test ear should be *masked*. Here, *white noise* is delivered to the non-test ear in order to occupy that cochlea and prevent the test tones (which may be transmitted from the test ear around or through the bony skull) being heard in the non-test ear.

Convention dictates that different symbols are used to depict left and right ears and also for air and bone conduction (Table 2.2).

TABLE 2.2 Symbols used in pure tone audiography

| CONDUCTION MEDIUM | LEFT | RIGHT |
|---|---|---|
| Air conduction | × | ○ |
| Bone conduction | ] | [ |

### The speech audiogram

The function of the inner ear is not only to detect the presence or absence of sound, but also to distinguish one sound from another in order to allow us to make sense of the sounds we hear. Some patients with a small sensorineural hearing loss (when tested with

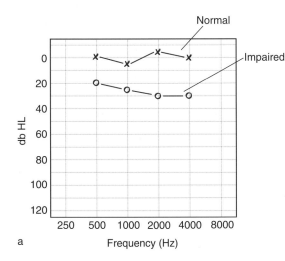

a

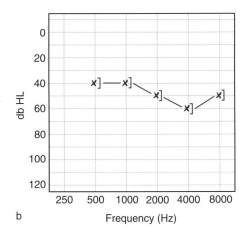

b

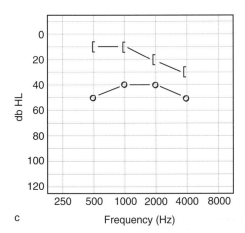

c

FIGURE 2.1 (a) Normal air conduction (left x) and impaired air conduction (right o). (b) Sensorineural impairment (left) (left air conduction x, left bone conduction ]). (c) Conductive impairment (right air conduction o, right-bone conduction []. For key to symbols see Table 2.2.

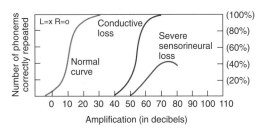

FIGURE 2.2 Speech audiometer.

pure tone audiometry) have great difficulty in understanding complex groups of sounds such as speech. The determination of this defect is the function of the speech audiogram.

Here a tape of spoken words is played to the patient and they are asked to repeat these words back to the tester. The percentage of correctly recognized words is recorded for various sound levels (Figure 2.2).

## Objective tests of hearing

### Electrical response audiometry

Here sounds in the form of clicks are presented to the ear and electrodes are used to pick up the resultant electrical responses which occur within the central nervous system auditory pathway. The electrical response can be measured at different points in this pathway.

In *electrocochleography*, a very fine-needle electrode is passed through the eardrum and allowed to rest on the promontory. This is the basal turn of the cochlea. The resulting electrical activity in the cochlea is recorded.

The electrical activity at the brainstem or cerebral cortex can also be measured by proper placement of skin electrodes. These electrical responses are known as *brainstem evoked responses* and *cortical evoked responses*, respectively. Analysis of the electrical responses can give an assessment of the hearing threshold. Also the pattern of the responses can suggest which part of the auditory pathway is affected in a sensorineural hearing loss.

### Otoacoustic emissions

Recently, it has been discovered that the ear as well as receiving sound, produces sounds! It is thought that these originate from the hair cells within the cochlea and that the sounds are generated as part of the process of transducing sound energy. The sound emissions generated can be measured using a small microphone placed in the ear and an averaging computer.

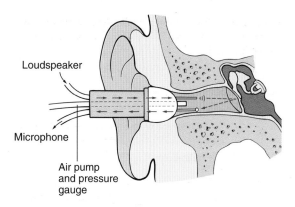

FIGURE 2.3 Tympanometer.

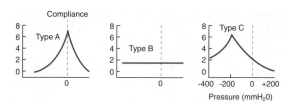

FIGURE 2.4 Tympanometry. Type A, normal. Type B, middle ear fluid. Type C, negative middle ear pressure.

Since these emissions are produced in response to sounds received by the cochlea, they may be employed as a useful test of cochlear function, and thus hearing. This technique is particularly useful as a screening test in neonates and young children since it is simple to perform, requires no cooperation from the patient and is non-invasive.

## Impedance audiometry (tympanometry)

This test measures the stiffness or compliance of the eardrum. A probe is inserted into the test ear. This probe has three channels (Figure 2.3), one to introduce sound, one to allow the pressure in the ear canal to be varied and one which carries a microphone which measures how much sound energy is reflected from the eardrum. Maximal sound energy passes through the eardrum when the pressure in the ear canal is the same as that in the middle ear. By varying the pressure in the ear canal and measuring the amount of sound reflected from the drum, the middle-ear pressure can be determined. The test produces a graph (Type A) whose peak coincides with the middle-ear pressure (Figure 2.4). A negative middle-ear pressure forces the peak to the left (Type C). Fluid in the middle ear produces a flat trace (Type B). An excessively tall peak indicates a hypermobile drum. Such a trace may occur in ossicular discontinuity.

## Stapedial reflexes

When the ear is exposed to a loud sound, the stapedius muscle reflexly contracts and dampens the vibrations of the ossicular chain in order to reduce the amount of sound energy transmitted and so protect the delicate inner ear. This stiffening of the ossic-

ular chain can be measured using the tympanometer. The presence or absence of this reflex, as well as the level of sound which elicits it, can be useful clinically. For example, in lesions of the facial nerve (which supplies the stapedius muscle as it passes through the middle ear), the presence of the stapedial reflex indicates that the lesion is distal to the branch which supplies the stapedius muscle. This helps to determine the site of the lesion. Also it can be used to give a crude indication of the hearing threshold. The reflex may be absent or reduced if there is a defect in the ossicular chain.

## Imaging in otology

Plain *X-rays* of the mastoid have been largely superseded by *computed tomography* (*CT*) scans, although some surgeons will still request them pre-operatively in mastoid surgery, since they do show the relationships of the important anatomical landmarks. Modern high-resolution CT scans of the temporal bone can show the details of the ossicles, cochlea, semicircular canals and mastoid system. In the evaluation of cholesteatoma, bone erosion is the most consistent sign (Figure 2.5).

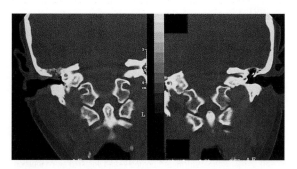

FIGURE 2.5 A cholesteatoma (left-hand image) filling the attic, with some erosion of the scutum – the outer attic wall.

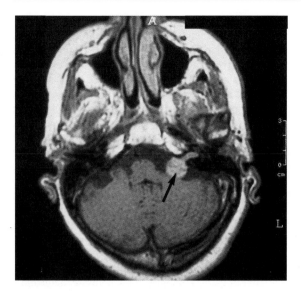

FIGURE 2.6 An MRI scan showing an acoustic neuroma extending into the internal auditory meatus and indenting the brainstem. Published with the kind permission of Mr C. Milford FRCS.

*MRI* scanning has become the primary investigation in the diagnosis of suspected acoustic neuromas (Figure 2.6). Other investigations, such as X-ray tomograms or CT scans, are largely obsolete.

# INVESTIGATIONS IN RHINOLOGY

## Tests of nasal function

### Air-flow measurements

Patients often complain of nasal obstruction and this is usually simple to assess on clinical examination. Therefore, formal testing of nasal air-flow is rarely performed in routine ENT practice. However, in some situations, such as in specialist rhinology, allergy clinics or in the research setting, such testing is performed.

*Peak inspiratory nasal air flow* can be measured using a modified peak flowmeter which has a mask which fits over the nose. Thus, effects of decongestants, allergens and drugs on nasal air flow can be assessed. *Acoustic rhinometry* is a technique which has only recently become available. As yet, it is primarily a research tool but may come into clinical practice as new applications for the technique are discovered. The basic principle is similar to that of underwater sonar. A sound click is shot into the nose and computer analysis of the resulting echo produces a trace which maps the contours and volume of the

nasal cavity. This technique does not directly measure air flow, but information concerning nasal patency can be inferred.

## Tests of ciliary function

The lining of the nose is covered with ciliated respiratory epithelium. It is important that these cilia function properly in order that secretions of the nasal cavity and sinuses are cleared. Both congenital and acquired conditions lead to such ciliary dysfunction.

The *saccharin taste test* is used to test the ciliary clearance of a fragment of saccharin placed on the anterior end of the inferior turbinate. Ciliary action passes the saccharin backwards and eventually it is deposited into the oropharynx, whereupon the patient first notices the sweet taste. A clearance time of more than 20 minutes is considered abnormal. It is important to ensure that the subject can in fact taste saccharin since a small number of normal people find this substance tasteless.

*Ciliary brushings* taken from the nasal cavity, and transported in an appropriate medium, can be examined with electron microscopy to reveal both the structure and beat frequency of the cilia. Abnormalities of either of these may lead to clinical disease.

## Tests of olfaction

Patients often complain of a lack of sense of smell (anosmia). Unfortunately, our clinical tests of a patient's olfactory ability are rather crude and these rarely give any useful additional information. A simple assessment can be achieved by asking the subject to sniff from *smell bottles* and name the product, e.g. coffee or lemon essence. A similar test is available commercially using scratch-and-sniff cards. Some work has been carried out recently on *cortical evoked response olfactometry*, but as yet this has failed to produce a clinically useful test of olfaction.

## Imaging in rhinology

Plain X-rays of the paranasal sinuses have been superseded by CT scanning which is universally available in the UK. CT scans demonstrate well the bony details of sinus anatomy and their relationship to important structures such as the orbit, optic nerve and base of skull (Figure 2.7). CT also shows bone destruction when it occurs with destructive lesions of the sinuses. However, CT does not depict soft tissues very well, and it can be particularly difficult to distinguish between retained secretions, thickened and oedema-

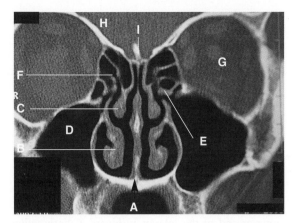

FIGURE 2.7 A CT scan of normal sinuses. Note the following structures: (a) nasal septum; (b) inferior turbinate; (c) middle turbinate; (d) maxillary sinus; (e) maxillary sinus ostium; (f) ethmoid sinuses; (g) orbit; (h) brain; (i) cribriform niche.

tous mucosa, polyps and tumour tissue. Despite these shortcomings, CT scanning has revolutionized our understanding of sinus disease and is an invaluable tool in investigation, diagnosis and planning of sinus operations.

# ALLERGY TESTING

Many patients with nasal symptoms have an underlying nasal allergy (allergic rhinitis). In order to reach a diagnosis and offer sensible allergen avoidance advice, allergy tests are frequently used.

## Skin testing

When positive, these tests confirm the production of IgE, which mediates this type of allergic reaction. A range of common potential allergens are tested by making a small scratch on the patient's forearm, then a drop of the allergen solution placed on top. The site is marked, and the process repeated for each allergen under test. After 20 minutes, the tests are read. A positive response is indicated by a weal-and-flare reaction.

Nearly all patients with seasonal allergic rhinitis show positive skin tests. Appropriately, however, such tests are limited by the fact that less than 50% of patients who have clinical features suggestive of perennial allergy have confirmatory skin tests. This may be because we have failed to test for the correct allergen, or possibly because a skin test assesses the presence of *systemic* IgE to various allergens. However, in allergic rhinitis, the main site of IgE production is in the *nose*, hence a positive skin test will only occur if the immunoglobulin has been absorbed into the general circulation. The presence of these circulating immunoglobulins can also be assessed at the serum level using the Radio-Allergo-Absorbent Test (RAST) blood test. This is no more accurate than skin testing, but is far more expensive.

## Investigation of neck lumps

See 'Investigation of neck lumps' in Chapter 8, page 82).

**KEY POINTS**
ENT Investigations

- The pure tone audiogram is a subjective test of hearing; here, 25 dB is the lower limit of normal hearing
- Objective tests of hearing are possible, but tend to be less accurate than subjective tests
- A flat tympanometry trace usually suggests a fluid-filled middle ear space
- MRI scanning is the best way to diagnose an acoustic neuroma
- CT scanning is the best way to image the sinuses
- Defects in the nasal airway are usually diagnosed on clinical examination
- Allergy tests can be helpful in advising patients with severe allergic rhinitis

# 3

# The mouth, tonsils and adenoids

Sore mouth and oral ulceration  18

Lumps and swellings in the mouth  21

Sore throat and tonsillitis  22

The adenoid, snoring and sleep apnoea  26

This chapter is organized in a problem-orientated fashion. This means that each section deals with one complaint with which a patient may present. As a result, there is some overlap of material. Nevertheless, this arrangement will make it easier to organize your thoughts when dealing with patients and any repetition will reinforce the important points.

The anatomy of the mouth and oral cavity is probably familiar to you and is summarized here in Figure 3.1.

---

## OVERVIEW
### Sore Mouth and Oral Ulceration

**Trauma**
- **Mechanical**, e.g. dentures
- **Chemical**, e.g. caustic, betel nut chewing

**Infective**
- **Viral**: herpes, measles, chickenpox, handfoot and mouth
- Bacterial: syphilis, scarlet fever, 'strawberry tongue'
- **Fungal**: Candida
- AIDS

**Haematological**
- Iron and folate deficiency anaemia
- Pernicious anaemia
- Agranulocytosis
- Polycythaemia

**Neoplastic**
- **Carcinoma**
- Leukaemia

**Autoimmune**
- Pemphigus
- Pemphigoid

**Idiopathic**
- **Aphthous ulcers**
- **Lichen planus**
- Behçet's syndrome
- Sarcoidosis
- Wegener's granulomatosis

**Others**
- Leukoplakia
- Vitamin C deficiency
- Black hairy tongue
- Stevens–Johnson syndrome

---

# SORE MOUTH AND ORAL ULCERATION

From the Overview, it is apparent that a large number of conditions may cause a sore or ulcerated mouth. Some of these are self-limiting and benign; others are malignant and life-threatening. We shall highlight the common and important conditions below. Many different diseases have similar presenting features such as an ulcer or pain in the mouth. Occasionally, patients may present with bleeding or discoloration within the oral cavity. Some conditions are simple to diagnose on their clinical appearance alone, whilst others may present a diagnostic challenge and a range of screening tests, including biopsy, may be required. An accurate history and examination are essential, taking particular note of the duration of the symptom, social/environmental factors such as smoking and alcohol consumption, as well as looking for signs and symptoms of systemic disease.

## Ulcers

### Traumatic ulcers

Acute traumatic ulcers are common, heal quickly and patients seldom seek medical advice. Chronic trauma, usually from ill-fitting dentures, often cause non-healing ulcers on the gums, lips or cheeks. Treatment is dental and entails refitting the dentures.

### Aphthous ulcers

These are common 'mouth ulcers'. They are small and painful ulcers which may occur singly or more often appear in crops. They usually affect the edge of the tongue, but can occur anywhere within the oral cavity. Their exact cause remains unknown although stress, poor diet, trauma, poor oral hygiene and hormonal changes have all been suggested. Usually, these ulcers present no more than a minor irritation for a few days before they resolve naturally. However, occasionally these ulcers are severe and recurrent and treatment should include simple analgesics and steroid pastels as well as excluding any potential causative factors.

Rarely, single, giant aphthous ulcers occur and here the diagnosis is often less certain; biopsy may be necessary.

### Infective ulcers

*Herpes simplex* mouth ulcers are painful and their appearances are similar to aphthous ulceration but

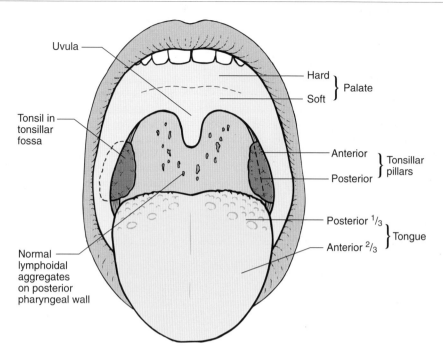

FIGURE 3.1 The anatomy of the mouth and oral cavity.

here mild pyrexia and malaise also occur. Acyclovir is effective if given in the early stages.

Rarely, immunocompromised or debilitated patients may develop patches of *herpes zoster* which affect the oral cavity following the distribution of the IXth and Xth cranial nerves.

The snail track ulcers of *syphilis* are classical, but rarely seen nowadays since more effective treatments for this condition have become available as is the severe ulceration of *trench mouth* which is caused by another spirochaete – Vincent's organism.

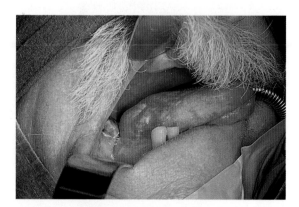

FIGURE 3.2 A pre-operative picture of a squamous cell carcinoma of the right lateral tongue border.

The oral manifestations of *AIDS* include oral candidiasis, tonsillitis, Kaposi's sarcoma and hairy leukoplakia of the tongue and in patients presenting with these conditions, one must have a high index of suspicion (see also Chapter 12, p. 152).

## Cancer (Figure 3.2)

Squamous cell carcinoma of the tongue and mouth nearly always starts as an ulcerating mass. These are progressive and painful, often with referred pain to the ear. They frequently arise in patients who are, or have been, heavy smokers and drinkers, spirits being particularly dangerous. Any ulcer which fails to heal within two weeks should be biopsied in order to exclude malignancy.

## Blood and dietary disorders

The haemopoietic agents iron, folate and vitamin $B_{12}$ are required for the maturation of healthy oral mucosa, and so deficiency of these factors is associated with oral ulceration. Other dietary deficiencies which cause a sore mouth include *pellagra* (deficiency of riboflavin and nicotinic acid) and *scurvy* with vitamin C deficiency. Polycythaemia, agranulocytosis and leukaemia can all cause oral ulceration.

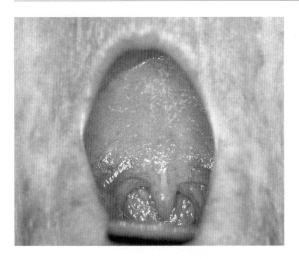

FIGURE 3.3 Oral *Candida* affecting the hard and soft palate.

# White patches in the mouth

### Candida (Figure 3.3)

Oral candidal infection tends to occur at the extremes of age and in the immunocompromised (e.g. diabetics and AIDS). *Candida* can occasionally occur on the palate as a result of steroid deposition with asthma inhalers. White specks coalesce to form patches or a membrane, which when lifted, reveals a red, raw, bleeding mucosal surface. The diagnosis is usually clinical and the condition responds to topical anti-fungicidal preparations, but if diagnostic doubt remains, scrapings of the lesion should be taken and submitted for microbiological examination.

### Leukoplakia (Figure 3.4)

A white patch in the mouth is called leukoplakia, although this is really only a descriptive term and not a diagnosis. The word 'leukoplakia' is often used to mean

hyperkeratosis of the oral mucosa. Hyperkeratosis is usually associated with local irritation, e.g. poorly fitting dentures, smoking, alcohol and strong spices. It is important to recognize and biopsy since 3% of such lesions will undergo malignant change within five years. In fact, erythroplakia (red patches in the mouth) have an even higher malignant potential. Even if such lesions prove benign on initial biopsy, regular review is recommended.

A particular form of this condition, called hairy leukoplakia (because of its histological appearances) occurs as white patches on the lateral border of the tongue in AIDS patients (see page 152).

## Lichen planus

This is an inflammatory disease, of unknown aetiology, which can affect the skin and oral cavity. The lesions are variable but may mimic hyperkeratosis. The classical form gives a white lace-like appearance. This condition may be extremely painful, but usually responds to local steroid preparations. If not, laser ablation is often effective.

## 'Black hairy tongue'

The cause of this condition is unknown but it does seem to be associated with smoking. There is an overgrowth of filiform papillae and treatment consists of vigorous brushing of the tongue in order to scrape these away (see Figure 3.5).

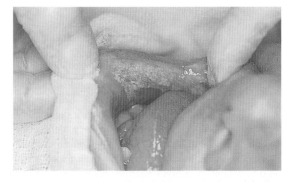

FIGURE 3.4 Leukoplakia affecting the inner surface of the lip.

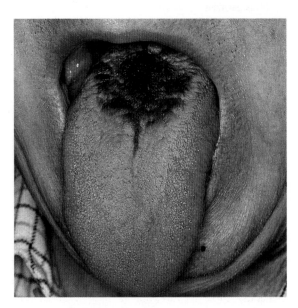

FIGURE 3.5 'Black Hairy Tongue'.

# LUMPS AND SWELLINGS IN THE MOUTH

**OVERVIEW**
Lumps and Swellings in the Mouth

**Congenital**
- Haemangioma
- Cystic hygroma

**Acquired**
- Ranula
- **Mucus retention cyst**
- Torus palatinus

**Neoplastic**
*Benign*
- Salivary tumours, e.g. pleomorphic adenoma

*Malignant*
- **Squamous cell carcinoma**
- Salivary tumours, e.g. adenoid cystic carcinoma
- Sarcomas
- Lymphomas

**Dental**
- **Abscess**
- Cyst

## Congenital masses

Generally, these are rare, but the most frequent congenital masses are haemangiomas and cystic hygromas

(see Chapter 8: Congenital Neck Remnants, pages 84-86). Any type of congenital oral mass may present at, or soon after, birth either with airway or feeding problems and later in life haemangiomas may present with bleeding. Treatment, where indicated, is via excision.

## Torus palitinus

This is a benign osteoma of the hard palate. Its surface may become ulcerated as a result of trauma from dentures, in which case the lesion may look malignant. These need only be removed if they cause symptoms or interfere with dentures.

## Mucus retention cysts

The mucosa of the oral cavity is rich in mucous glands. Should these become blocked, a retention cyst develops. These smooth, pale, round swellings may occur anywhere in the mouth or lips. Excision is only required if they are symptomatic or the diagnosis is uncertain.

## Ranula

A ranula (which literally means 'small frog') is a retention cyst which forms in the floor of the mouth under the tongue. It develops from the submandibular or sublingual gland ducts. The swelling may enlarge and reduce intermittently as the contents discharge and then re-accumulate. Marsupialization (stitching open) of the cyst is the most effective treatment.

## Oral cavity tumours

Both benign and malignant tumours may affect the oral cavity and present as a lump in the mouth. The intra-oral minor salivary glands may give rise to a variety of tumours, e.g. a benign pleomorphic adenoma or malignant adenoid cystic carcinoma. Also, lymphomas may affect the tonsil. However, the commonest oral cavity tumour is a squamous cell carcinoma.

### Squamous cell carcinomas (Figure 3.6)

These tend to occur in mid to late life. Here alcohol and tobacco are strong aetiological factors. They may arise from areas of leuko- or erythroplakia. The commonest sites are the lateral border of the tongue and floor of mouth. The patient will commonly complain of a sore throat, pain, referred otalgia, and sometimes bleeding

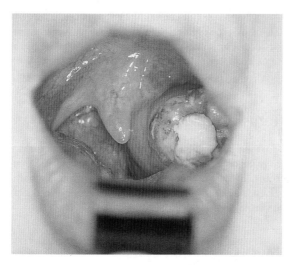

FIGURE 3.6 Carcinoma of the tonsil.

or difficulty in swallowing. These cancers spread to nearby lymph nodes and a lump in the neck may be the presenting feature. A deep peroral biopsy is essential, not only in order to confirm the diagnosis, but also to assess the depth of invasion of the tumour which has a considerable bearing on the prognosis. Therefore, this procedure should not be performed in the outpatient department, but in the operating theatre under general anaesthesia where an adequately sized sample may be taken and full pan-endoscopy performed.

Pan-endoscopy includes examination of the whole of the upper aerodigestive tract. This is vital since a proportion of patients with one primary tumour in this area will, in fact, already have a second primary malignancy. Obviously, this must be identified and treated appropriately if the patient is to have any chance of survival.

Treatment options include both external beam and interstitial radiotherapy, as well as surgical *en bloc* resection of the tumour with all affected hard and soft tissues. The surgically created defect will need reconstruction in order to give both a cosmetically and functionally acceptable result.

**KEY POINTS**
## Features of Oral Cavity Cancers

- Smoking and alcohol are aetiological factors
- Most often present with a painful ulcerating mass
- May present with referred otalgia
- Spread by lymph to local neck nodes
- Early treatment of small cancers offers the best hope of any cure

Great advances in oral cavity reconstructive techniques have been made recently with the advent of myocutaneous free flaps, e.g. radial forearm flap. Here a part of the radius may also be incorporated into the flap in order to reconstruct a bony mandibular defect.

Chemotherapy may have some role to play but only in the palliation of symptoms. In small tumours which have no nodal spread, the five-year survival is approximately 30%; in more advanced disease, the outlook is even more miserable.

# SORE THROAT AND TONSILLITIS

**OVERVIEW**
## Sore Throat and Tonsillitis

**Trauma**
- **Chemical: environmental exposure**
- **Alcohol**
- **Cigarettes**
- **Gastric acid**

**Infections**
- **Viral pharyngitis**
- **Bacterial tonsillitis**
- **Quinsy**
- **Glandular fever**
- Candida
- **Infection secondary to purulent postnasal drip**

**Tumours**
- **Squamous cell carcinoma**
- Lymphoma

The common causes of sore throat may be broadly classified as traumatic, infective and neoplastic. It is usually obvious from the history and examination into which category the patient falls. In cases of chronic sore throat, one must exclude the non-specific causes of pharyngeal trauma, namely, tobacco smoke, alcohol, gastro-oesophageal reflux, environmental factors such as dust or fumes and postnasal drip secondary to rhinosinusitis (Figure 3.7).

## Infective pharyngitis

All of us have suffered, at some time or another, from a sore throat. The vast majority of these are due to infective viral pharyngitis, which in most cases is triv-

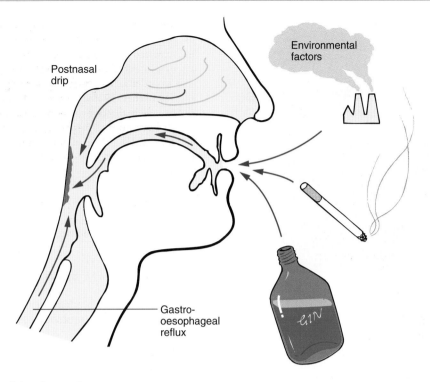

Postnasal
drip

Environmental
factors

Gastro-
oesophageal
reflux

FIGURE 3.7 Causes of chronic sore throat.

ial and self-limiting. The usual agents are influenza, parainfluenza, rhino- and adenoviruses; however, herpes simplex and zoster viruses are also less commonly implicated.

Other organisms causing sore throat include beta-haemolytic *Streptococcus*, *Pneumococcus* and *Haemophilus influenzae*. Much less commonly, oral gonorrhoea, syphilis and tuberculosis may occur.

Oral candidiasis is uncommon in otherwise healthy individuals, and this condition must alert one to the possibility of an underlying immunosuppressive disease such as AIDS.

## Tonsillitis (Figure 3.8)

The diagnosis of tonsillitis is usually not in doubt from the history and clinical findings. The features of tonsillitis include:

- Sore throat
- Difficulty in swallowing
- Pyrexia
- General malaise
- Halitosis
- Lymphadenopathy
- Exudative inflammation
- Enlargement of the tonsils

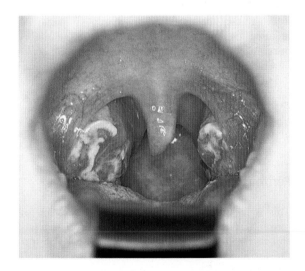

FIGURE 3.8 Bacterial tonsillitis.

This so-called acute *follicular* tonsillitis is common and is usually caused by B haemolytic *Streptococcus*, *Pneumococcus* or *Haemophilus influenzae*; sometimes this occurs secondary to an initial viral infection.

A similar clinical picture can accompany glandular fever, but here the tonsils are covered in a white/grey exudate (Figure 3.9) and generalized lymphadenopathy

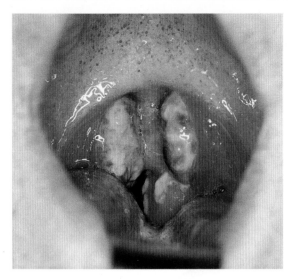

FIGURE 3.9 The tonsils in glandular fever.

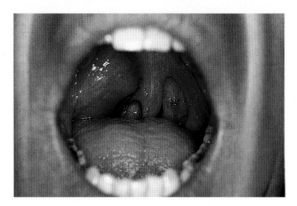

FIGURE 3.10 A quinsy. Note how the uvula is pushed towards the unaffected side.

sometimes with hepatosplenomegaly may occur. However, firm diagnosis of this condition usually requires a Paul Bunnell or monospot test. Treatment in mild cases may simply consist of bed rest, simple analgesia and oral fluid replacement. In more severe cases antibiotics, such as penicillin or erythromycin, may be required. In very severe cases, where the patient is unable to take adequate fluid orally, admission may be required for intravenous fluid replacement and antibiotics.

Complications of acute tonsillitis are rare nowadays. However, febrile convulsions may occur in children and infection may spread to form an abscess in one of the potential spaces between fascial planes in the neck, namely peritonsillar (quinsy), parapharyngeal and retropharyngeal spaces.

## Peritonsillar abscess or quinsy (Figure 3.10)

This is the most common infective complication of tonsillitis. Here the infection spreads to the tissues lateral to the tonsil, and an abscess develops. The features of a quinsy include the following.

- Due to the laterally based swelling, the tonsil is pushed medially.
- There is characteristic displacement of the uvula from the midline and towards the unaffected side.
- These patients are generally more unwell than with simple tonsillitis.
- Drooling and fetor occur.
- Trismus (pain on opening the mouth) is a prominent feature due to inflammation of the pterygoid muscles.

Treatment consists in decompression of the abscess either by aspiration or inscision (Figure 3.11). This leads to instant symptomatic relief and the condition resolves quickly with antibiotics.

## Indications for tonsillectomy

The indications for tonsillectomy may be absolute or relative. The absolute indications are:

- suspected malignancy
- as part of another procedure, e.g. uvulopharyngo-palatoplasty (UPPP)
- children with obstructive sleep apnoea syndrome (OSAS)

The relative indications are:

- recurrent acute tonsillitis
- chronic tonsillitis
- previous quinsy (once or twice previously)
- febrile convulsions

As far as the relative indications are concerned, most ENT surgeons would consider three attacks of tonsillitis a year for two consecutive years, or five attacks in one year as sufficient to warrant tonsillectomy. Having said this, it must be appreciated that each case should be assessed individually. For example, one may well consider tonsillectomy in a child who has had only two attacks of tonsillitis but each associated with a febrile convulsion, or a student, who may not as yet meet the above criteria, but who is entering an important academic year and cannot afford time away from their studies.

The size of the tonsils has little to do with their disease status. Small tonsils can be just as troublesome as large ones. However in the case of patients who suffer with obstructive sleep apnoea syndrome (OSAS; see pages 27–30) large tonsils should be removed, even if they are otherwise healthy.

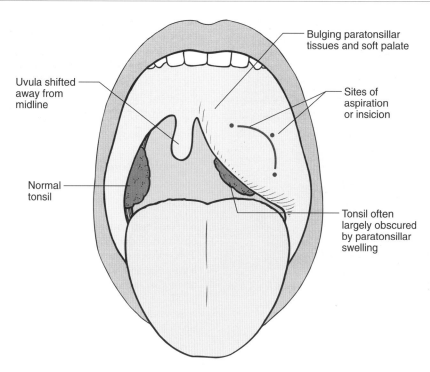

Bulging paratonsillar tissues and soft palate

Uvula shifted away from midline

Sites of aspiration or insicion

Normal tonsil

Tonsil often largely obscured by paratonsillar swelling

FIGURE 3.11 The appearance of a quinsy showing the sites for aspiration or incision.

## Tonsillectomy

This is one of the most commonly performed operations in the UK. The patient is usually required to stay for one night postoperatively in order that any bleeding may be recognized and dealt with. Nowadays, the tonsils are dissected and removed. However, previously a tonsillar guillotine was commonly used. Haemostasis is usually achieved with diathermy or ligatures. After the tonsils have been removed, the tonsillar fossae become coated with a layer of whitish, fibrinous exudate, which is sometimes mistakenly thought to represent an infection (Figure 3.12).

The pharynx has a rich nerve supply and so the operation site is often extremely painful. Referred otalgia is also common and regular simple analgesia is usually required.

Bleeding is the most serious and most common complication of tonsillectomy. Bleeding can occur in the first few hours after the operation (*reactionary haemorrhage*) as a result of a slipped ligature or inadequate haemostasis. This may require a return to theatre. A so-called *secondary haemorrhage* occurs as a result of a postoperative infection, usually 5–10 days after the operation. The patient should be admitted and the bleeding will invariably stop with intravenous antibiotics; rarely surgical haemostasis is required.

Postoperatively, the patient should be encouraged to eat and drink as normal. The old-fashioned jelly and ice-cream diet has now been replaced with crisps, biscuits and toast, since it is believed that the process of chewing after tonsillectomy is important in speeding recovery and also helps to prevent postoperative infection.

### KEY POINTS
### Sore Throat, Tonsillitis and Tonsillectomy

- In patients with chronic sore throat, exclude any provoking factors
- Glandular fever can cause similar clinical appearances to tonsillitis
- Recurrent tonsillitis and OSAS in children are the common indications for tonsillectomy
- Bleeding is the commonest complication of tonsillectomy
- Bleeding at 5–10 days after tonsillectomy represents an infection of the surgical site
- After tonsillectomy, patients should be encouraged to eat and drink as normal

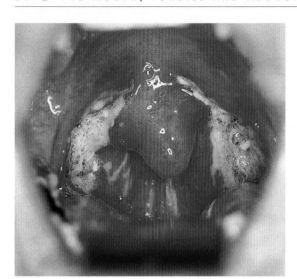

FIGURE 3.12 The normal appearance of the tonsillar fossa in the first few days following tonsillectomy.

# THE ADENOID, SNORING AND SLEEP APNOEA

## The adenoid

### What is the adenoid? (Figure 3.13)

The adenoid is a collection of loosely arranged, non-encapsulated, lymphoid tissue which lies at the back of

the nose or postnasal space and is attached to the posterior wall of the nasopharynx. There is only one adenoid; despite this, one will often hear doctors and patients alike refer to the 'adenoids'. The size of the adenoid gradually increases from birth until the age of 6 years; after this, atrophy occurs and most children will have no significant adenoid tissue after the age of 12 years.

## Adenoidal conditions (Figure 3.14)

### Nasal

An enlarged adenoid may cause childhood nasal obstruction due to blockage of the posterior choanae. This may give the voice a nasal quality, induce mouth breathing and also interfere with eating. The child often also suffers with a runny nose since the normal nasal secretions are not sufficiently cleared from the nose. If the adenoid should become infected, the anterior rhinorrhoea may become profuse and offensive. Children with enlarged adenoids often snore and, in combination with big tonsils, may sufficiently narrow the upper airways as to cause obstructive sleep apnoea syndrome (OSAS). This is discussed in more detail below.

### Otological

The adenoid, if enlarged or infected, may compromise the function of the eustachian tube and this can result

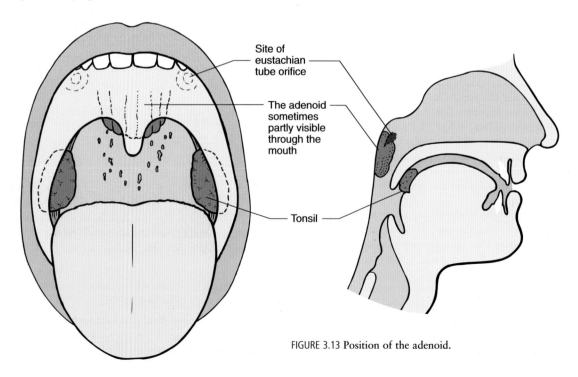

FIGURE 3.13 Position of the adenoid.

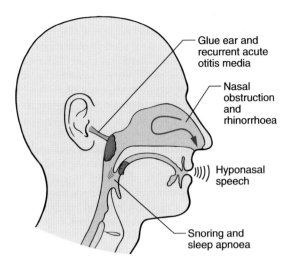

FIGURE 3.14 Adenoidal conditions.

in secretory otitis media (glue ear). A chronically infected adenoid may allow ascending infections to reach the middle ear via the eustachian tube. This may lead to repeated attacks of acute otitis media.

## Diagnosis

The diagnosis of adenoidal disease is usually suspected clinically from the features described above. Confirmatory examination of the postnasal space is difficult in most children since they will not often tolerate an oral mirror or nasal endoscope, and in difficult diagnostic cases a lateral soft-tissue X-ray (Figure 3.15) of the postnasal space will often demonstrate the adenoid. However, the diagnosis is established by examination and finger palpation of the postnasal space under general anaesthesia.

## Adenoidectomy

The adenoid is blindly curetted under general anaesthesia. The most significant risk is that of bleeding. This can occur at the time of surgery or soon after, in which case this is termed a 'reactionary haemorrhage'; if severe, this may require insertion of a postnasal space pack.

Postoperatively, the adenoid bed may occasionally become infected and then bleeding can occur. This is termed a 'secondary haemorrhage' and usually presents at 5–10 days. The bleeding nearly always settles with bed rest, observation and antibiotics. The procedure is not painful (unlike tonsillectomy), and when performed in isolation or with grommet insertion, is frequently carried out as a day case.

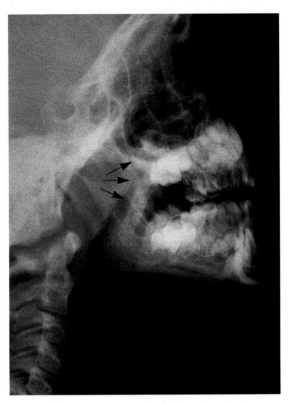

FIGURE 3.15 X-ray of an adenoid. Note the narrowing of the posterior nasal airway due to the enlarged adenoid.

The soft palate acts as a type of flap valve and functionally separates the nasal and oral cavities. In patients who have a short or abnormal palate, the adenoid may contribute to the effective functioning of this valve. Here, adenoidectomy should be avoided because there is a significant risk of producing palatal incompetence which results in nasal regurgitation of liquids and nasal escape during speech (rhinolalia-aperta or hypernasality).

## Snoring and sleep apnoea

Snoring and the obstructive type of sleep apnoea syndrome (OSAS) are described together since all patients who have OSAS snore. Remember, however, that not all patients who snore suffer from OSAS. Patients who are on the borderline of developing OSAS may be tipped into the full-blown state with the ingestion of alcohol or other sedatives.

## Definitions

*Snoring* is the noise produced in sleep by the vibration of the soft tissues of the pharynx, such as the soft palate and tongue base.

*Sleep apnoea* is defined as thirty or more episodes of cessation of breathing each with a minimum duration of 10 seconds, occurring over a 7-hour period of sleep.

*Obstructive sleep apnoea.* Here the apnoea is due to upper airways collapse. As a result, the chest movements continue in an effort to shift air through the obstructed segment. With time, the blood oxygen saturation level falls and when critically low levels are reached, a central reflex is activated which causes the patient to waken slightly and take a deep breath in order to overcome the obstruction. Long term, these periods of desaturation may lead to pulmonary hypertension and right ventricular strain, which may lead to ventricular failure, and finally cor pulmonale.

*Central sleep apnoea.* This is less common than the obstructive type and here the central respiratory drive is at fault. Such patients should be referred to a neurologist.

*Sleep apnoea index.* This is the number of apnoeic periods per hour.

## Signs and symptoms of OSAS

Adult patients will often be overweight with a large neck and frequently overindulge in alcohol. Full ENT examination is essential, paying special attention to the likely sites of upper airway obstruction (Figure 3.16). In children, the syndrome occurs almost without exception in conjunction with adenotonsillar hypertrophy. Snoring is the cardinal symptom and the patient's partner will often give this history. Occasionally, they will also describe the classical sequence of events: the patient stops breathing for a period, they appear to be struggling for breath, and at times will become agitated with movements of their limbs, etc.; eventually, the obstruction is overcome with a loud gasp and intake of breath. This poor quality sleep leads to daytime sleepiness and lethargy, a feeling of waking unrefreshed, as well as poor concentration and memory and loss of libido. In the later stages, the medical complications due to heart failure may become apparent.

## Investigation of snoring and OSAS

In order to establish whether the patient is suffering with simple snoring or OSAS, a *sleep study* should be performed. Here, the patient is admitted to a sleep unit overnight and various parameters are measured. These include pulse, ECG, oxygen saturation, chest and abdominal movements, and audio and video tape in order to listen to the snoring and observe the patient's body movements during sleep.

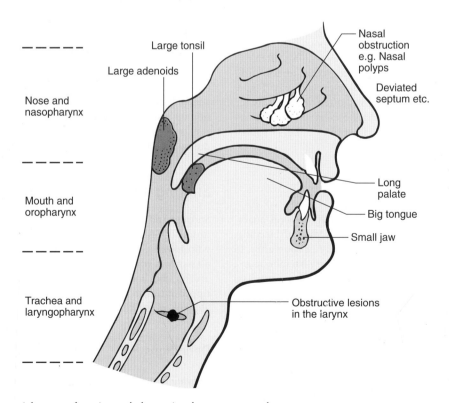

FIGURE 3.16 Potential causes of snoring and obstructive sleep apnoea syndrome.

*Sleep nasendoscopy* is performed in order to identify the site of the vibration in snoring, or the site of the upper airway obstruction in OSAS. Here, the patient is sedated and sleep is induced. A flexible nasendoscope is introduced via the nose and the upper airways visualized directly.

A suggestion as to the site of the obstruction may be obtained in the outpatient department by introducing a flexible endoscope to visualize the airway then pinching the nose in order to produce an air-tight seal. The patient is instructed to perform a forced reverse Valsalva; this is known as the *Mueller manoeuvre*.

## Management of snoring and OSAS

### Lifestyle

It is vital to encourage the obese patient to lose weight since, if successful, this will often have a dramatic effect on their symptoms as well as improving their health generally. Similarly, alcohol consumption must be brought to within sensible limits and other sedatives should be withdrawn.

### Medical

In patients with OSAS, medications designed to reduce the amount of rapid eye movement (REM) sleep, which is the period of sleep most likely to produce OSAS, or respiratory stimulants may be effective therapy.

Continuous positive airway pressure (CPAP) ventilation is an effective treatment for OSAS. This involves wearing a mask over the nose, introducing air under pressure. This then acts as a pneumatic splint and helps to keep the upper airways open and so prevent collapse. The generating pump can be noisy and the mask uncomfortable. As a result, this treatment may be poorly tolerated by some patients.

## Surgery

In virtually all children, snoring is reduced and OSAS cured by adenotonsillectomy. In adults, any surgical treatment must be aimed at the portion of the airways which is responsible for the vibration or collapse. Obstructions in the nose such as nasal polyps or a deviated nasal septum are generally simple to deal with. If the soft palate or lateral pharyngeal bands are the source of the problem, surgical resection may be effective; this is known as a uvulopharyngopalatoplasty (UPPP) (Figure 3.17).

Various types of less radical palatal procedures have been described for snoring, for example laser palatal scarring. The rationale here is to induce fibro-

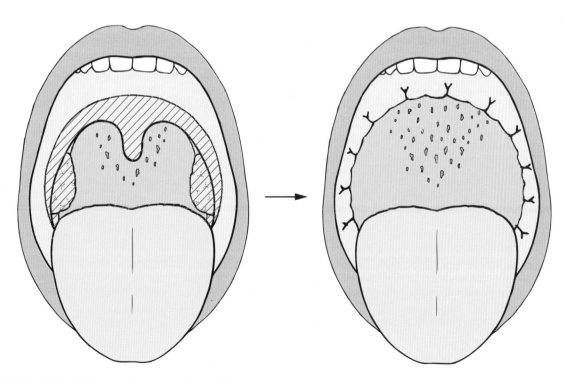

FIGURE 3.17 The UPPP operation for snoring and sleep apnoea.

sis in the soft palate, which now being stiffer, is less likely to vibrate as a result of air flow across it.

Tongue base collapse is far more difficult to treat surgically. Major jaw and hyoid advancements have been described, but these are probably best reserved for those patients who have congenitally small mandibles (micrognathia). A tracheostomy is an effective treatment since it bypasses the obstructed segment of the airway and abolishes OSAS completely. This is reserved for extreme cases which are unresponsive to other forms of treatment.

## KEY POINTS
### Snoring and OSAS

- Snoring is the cardinal symptom of OSAS, but not all snorers have OSAS
- OSAS can have major cardiorespiratory effects
- A history of the patient's nocturnal symptoms should be taken from their partner
- Weight loss and other lifestyle improvements is often effective therapy
- Any nasal condition which reduces air flow, such as polyps or deviated nasal septum, should be treated
- Sleep study is required in order to confirm the diagnosis of OSAS
- Sleep nasendoscopy helps to determine the site of snoring and obstruction in OSAS

## CASE STUDY

Thomas is 89 years old and twenty years ago was treated with radium needles for a small carcinoma on the right side of his tongue. He made a good recovery from this, and after five years was discharged from further follow up. He now complains of pain in the right side of his tongue and also of some right-sided earache. On examination, there is a hard 2-cm swelling extending to the right lateral tongue border with some ulceration on its surface. There is nothing else to find on examination.

1 What is the most likely diagnosis?
2 How would you confirm this?
3 What are the risk factors of oral cavity carcinomas?

**Comments**
1 Squamous cell carcinoma.
2 Biopsy is essential, preferably under general anaesthetic, where a deep biopsy can be taken and some assessment made as to the depth of the tumour. Also pan-endoscopy should be performed in order to exclude a second primary tumour.
3 In this case, the greatest risk factor is the previous radiotherapy. It is unlikely that he has recurrent disease after twenty years. It is far more likely that his current tumour is radiotherapy induced. Other risk factors are smoking, betel nut and other strong spice chewing, chronic dental trauma and alcoholism. Remember that leukoplakia and erythroplakia are premalignant conditions.

# 4

# The salivary glands

Structure and function of the salivary glands  32

Innervation of the salivary glands  33

Diseases of the salivary glands  34

Surgery of the salivary glands  36

# STRUCTURE AND FUNCTION OF THE SALIVARY GLANDS

There are three main paired salivary glands: the parotid, the submandibular and the sublingual. There is also a large number of tiny minor salivary glands scattered around the oral cavity and the oropharynx. Their function is to provide lubrication for the oral mucosa and begin the digestion of food. Their secretions also have an antibacterial function. They are reflexly stimulated to produce saliva and they may secrete up to 1 litre in 24 hours.

## The parotid gland (Figure 4.1)

This is the largest of the paired salivary glands. It is a serous gland producing a watery saliva. It is situated in the cheek lying in the space between the mastoid process and the mandible. Deeply lies the styloid process, its attached musculature and the carotid sheath. Laterally the gland is flat, covered by the thick parotid fascia, lying close to the skin. The parotid secretions drain into the mouth via the parotid duct which opens at the level of the second upper molar tooth.

The facial nerve emerges from the stylomastoid foramen that lies at the posterior/deep border of the gland. As it passes through the gland, it divides into five branches which supply the muscles of the face. The facial nerve divides the gland into deep and superficial parts. It is the structure most at risk during parotid surgery. Also lying within the deep lobe of the parotid is the last part of the external carotid artery as it follows its tortuous course, together with the retromandibular vein and several parotid lymph nodes that drain the surrounding area.

## The submandibular gland (Figure 4.2)

This is a mixed serous and mucous gland that lies in a triangular space bounded by the mylohyoid muscle, the mandible and roofed by the deep cervical fascia that is attached to the mandible and hyoid bones. The gland is made up of a large superficial lobe that lies on the mylohyoid muscle and a deep lobe that wraps around the free posterior edge of the muscle to lie in the floor of the mouth. The submandibular duct (Wharton's duct) runs forward from the deep lobe to open into the mouth as a papilla next to the frenulum of the tongue. Three important nerves are related to the gland. They are the hypoglossal and lingual nerves, that are associated with the deep lobe and duct, the third being the marginal mandibular branch of the facial nerve running just under the skin overlying the gland. A number of submandibular lymph nodes lie close to, and also within, the gland.

## The sublingual gland

This is the smallest of the paired glands and lies in the floor of the mouth along the course of the submandibular duct. It is oblong in shape and is mucussecreting. It drains by 10–15 small ducts either directly into the mouth or into the submandibular duct. Its relations are similar to those of the deep lobe of the submandibular gland.

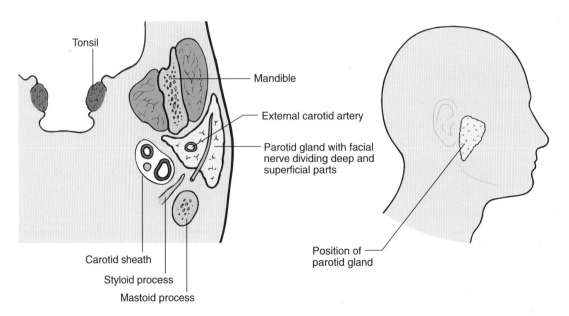

Tonsil

Mandible

External carotid artery

Parotid gland with facial nerve dividing deep and superficial parts

Carotid sheath

Styloid process

Mastoid process

Position of parotid gland

FIGURE 4.1 Transverse section through the parotid gland showing its anatomical relationships.

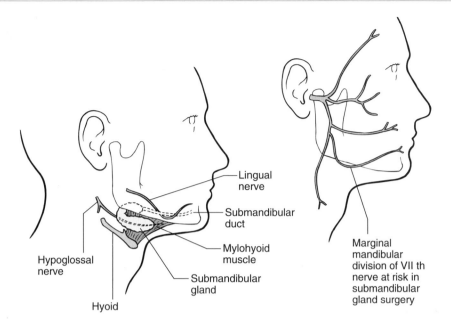

FIGURE 4.2 The submandibular gland and its anatomical relations.

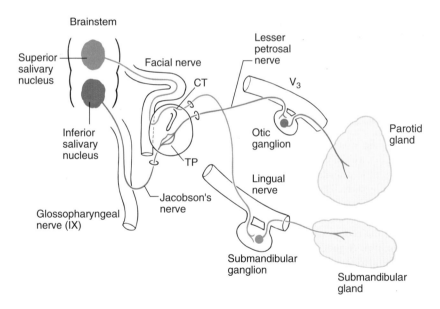

FIGURE 4.3 Diagrammatic representation of the nerve supply to the parotid and submandibular glands. CT = chorda tympani; TP = tympanic plexus.

# INNERVATION OF THE SALIVARY GLANDS (Figure 4.3)

The innervation of the salivary glands follows a complex course. The parotid is supplied by the inferior salivary nucleus of the brainstem. Secretormotor fibres travel with the IXth cranial nerve, leaving this at its exit from the base of the skull to ascend as Jacobson's nerve into the middle ear cleft. From here, the fibres exit the ear and travel into the floor of the middle cranial fossa as the lesser petrosal nerve to join the mandibular division of the trigeminal nerve. This leaves the skull through the foramen ovale and the fibres then reach the parotid via the auriculotemporal branch of the mandibular division of the trigeminal nerve ($V_3$).

The submandibular and sublingual glands are supplied by the superior salivary nucleus. Fibres travel with the facial nerve, then branch off as the chorda tympani. This leaves the VIIth within the middle ear cleft, to exit into the infratemporal fossa, where it joins the lingual nerve to reach the glands. The chorda tympani also supplies the sensation of taste to the anterior two-thirds of the tongue but via different fibres.

> **KEY POINTS**
> ## Innervation of the Salivary Glands
>
> - The facial nerve, which supplies the muscles of the face, traverses the parotid, and divides into its five main branches within the gland substance
> - The parotid gland has a dense capsule which is painful when stretched
> - The submandibular gland and duct are closely related to the hypoglossal (XIIth) and the lingual (a branch of the mandibular division of the trigeminal nerve). The marginal mandibular branch of the facial nerve runs just under the skin which overlies the submandibular gland

# DISEASES OF THE SALIVARY GLANDS

The salivary glands may be affected by a range of disease processes. Disease may be limited to a single gland, but there are systemic disorders that may affect a number, or all, of the glands. The two main symptoms that may arise from disease of the salivary glands are swelling and pain. If the glandular dysfunction is widespread, dryness of the mouth can result, but this is a less common symptom. A good history is vital to elicit which glands are affected, the duration of the symptoms and whether there are any indications of a systemic disease. Conditions which affect the salivary glands can also affect the lacrimal gland and so the patient should also be questioned for symptoms of dry, itchy eyes or swelling of the lacrimal sac.

Examination should include inspection and palpation of all the salivary glands both externally and intra-orally, using bimanual palpation. The oral cavity and oropharynx should be examined (rarely, deep lobe parotid tumours can present as a swelling in the oropharynx) as well as the neck, and if indicated, the rest of the body. It is important to also examine the integrity of the facial nerve. Facial nerve palsy due to a parotid swelling should raise the suspicion of a malignant lesion.

The list of diseases shown below is not all inclusive, but the more common and important conditions are discussed in more detail.

> **OVERVIEW**
> ## Diseases of the Salivary Glands
>
> **Congenital**
> Cysts
> Vascular malformations, e.g. haemangiomas
>
> **Acquired**
> Infective/inflammatory
> **Sialolithiasis**
> **Sialadenitis**
>   acute/chronic
>   bacterial/viral
>   systemic viral infections, e.g. mumps, HIV
>   granulomatous diseases, e.g. TB, sarcoidosis
>   actinomycosis
> Autoimmune
>   Sjögren's syndrome
>   Drugs
>   Oral contraceptives
>   Thiouracil
>   Neoplastic
>   Benign
>     cysts
>     **pleomorphic adenoma**
>     **Warthin's tumour**
>     oncocytoma
>     lipoma
>     haemangioma
>   Malignant
>     **mucoepidermoid**
>     **adenoidcystic**
>     acinic cell
>     adenocarcinoma

## Systemic viral infections

Mumps, caused by the paramyxovirus, is the commonest cause of bilateral parotid gland enlargement. The submandibular glands can be involved, but this is rare. It occurs mainly in children. The usual signs consist of systemic upset, swelling and pain which is due to the stretching of the parotid capsule. Infection with the human immunodeficiency virus (HIV) can be associated with enlargement of the major salivary glands.

## Sialadenitis

Acute infection of either the parotid or submandibular gland presents with pain and a swollen gland. Acute parotitis commonly occurs in older, debilitated patients, who may be dehydrated and have poor oral hygiene. It can be seen in the community or sometimes in debilitated hospital patients, e.g. after major surgery. The local symptoms may be associated with pyrexia and systemic upset. On examination, the gland is swollen and tender, and there may be pus visible coming from the opening of the parotid duct in the mouth. In the case of the submandibular gland, the tissues of the floor of the mouth are often swollen and oedematous. Treatment is with high-dose antibiotics, rehydration and oral hygiene. Citrus mouthwashes will also improve saliva flow. Untreated, a parotid abscess may occur and this necessitates surgical drainage.

Chronic sialadenitis with recurring inflammation and pain may follow an acute infection or begin insidiously. Pain and swelling in episodes or transiently after meals are common symptoms. There are chronic changes and scarring in the architecture of the gland. Treatment of the acute episodes with antibiotics is helpful. The submandibular gland is most often affected and on occasions only surgical excision will remove the symptoms.

## Sialolithiasis

This describes the formation of stones (calculi) within the salivary glands and often occurs in combination with chronic sialadenitis. Most salivary calculi occur within the submandibular gland, possibly because of its thicker, more calcium-rich secretions, but they can occur in the parotid. Calculi usually present with postprandial swelling and pain in the gland, or in association with repeated infections. On examination, the gland may be tender and swollen, and if the calculi have migrated into the submandibular duct, they may be palpated in the floor of the mouth. X-ray of the area may show the calculi and injection of the gland via its duct with radio-opaque dye (a sialogram) will also illustrate these and the usual associated changes of chronic sialadenitis. Initial treatment is conservative, with oral fluids and sialogogues (such as lemon drops) as sometimes small stones may pass spontaneously. But if the situation becomes more problematic, the stone(s) can either be surgically excised from the duct or the gland itself removed.

## Granulomatous disease

Tuberculosis can involve the intraparotid lymph nodes, or rarely affect the gland itself. In children, non-tuberculous mycobacterial infections are sometimes seen as a cold abscess of the lymph nodes adjacent to the submandibular or parotid glands.

## Sjögren's syndrome

This syndrome affects many organ systems and is probably due to an autoimmune cause. Xerostomia (dry mouth) and keratoconjunctivitis sicca (dry eyes) are characteristic. A large number of these patients will have parotid gland enlargement, which is usually diffuse. Minor and major salivary glands are affected by the disease which leads to a reduced saliva flow and therefore xerostomia. Diagnosis is made by biopsy of the oral mucosa, usually on the inner lip. Treatment is symptomatic.

## Neoplastic disease

Neoplastic disease of the salivary glands is uncommon; 80–90% of salivary neoplasms arise in the parotid gland and a similar proportion of these will be benign in nature. Tumours arising in the submandibular or the minor glands are uncommon but are much more likely to be malignant. Investigations include fine-needle aspiration (FNA) of the mass, sialography and sometimes computed tomography. FNA may be helpful, but when the exact diagnosis is still in doubt, excision biopsy of the gland may be needed. Incisional biopsies should not be undertaken as there is a risk of seeding tumour and thus tumour recurrence.

### Benign tumours

Benign neoplastic tumours classically present as slow-growing, painless masses. The patient may have noticed a small mass for some time and only seek help when it becomes more noticeable (Figure 4.4). Facial or other nerve palsy does not tend to occur. Examination usually reveals a smooth, subcutaneous swelling with no attachment to skin.

Pleomorphic adenomas are the most common of salivary gland tumours and usually arise in the parotid. They are benign, but if they are present for many years, malignant change may occur. Treatment is by surgical excision, taking care to remove it completely and to include a cuff of normal parotid tissue around the palpable lump. Care must be taken not to spill tumour cells as these can cause recurrences. Warthin's tumour or adenolymphoma (which is not malignant, despite its name) also tend to arise in the parotid. It is most commonly found in the tail of the parotid and usually occurs in older men; occasionally

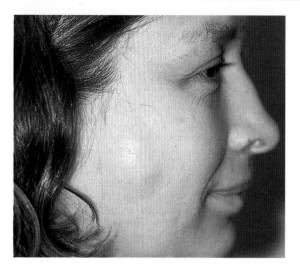

FIGURE 4.4 A pleomorphic adenoma of the parotid gland. In this case the mass is quite anterior.

it occurs bilaterally (see Figure 4.5). Treatment is by excision.

### Malignant tumours

Malignant salivary neoplasms are relatively uncommon. Symptoms include a rapidly growing swelling, often with pain and the involvement of other structures. Facial nerve palsy with a parotid tumour is almost diagnostic of malignancy. Local lymph node metastases may occur and so the neck must be included in the examination. Malignant tumours are more common in the sublingual and minor salivary glands than in the parotid. Therefore, swellings in these areas

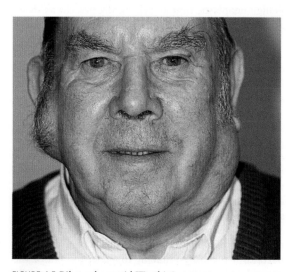

FIGURE 4.5 Bilateral parotid Warthin's tumours.

must be treated with a higher index of suspicion. Minor salivary glands are dispersed throughout the oral and nasal cavities. As a result, minor salivary gland tumours may occur anywhere within these areas.

Muco-epidermoid tumours have a range of malignancy, from low to high. Treatment depends on tumour grade; low-grade tumours can be treated with excision alone, but high-grade lesions may need radical resection and radiotherapy.

Adenoid cystic carcinoma is the commonest salivary gland malignancy. This tumour grows gradually and local spread may be extensive, often with infiltration along nerves which may produce 'skip lesions'. Treatment is by radical local excision with radiotherapy. Patients may live with their disease for some years, but the long-term prognosis is poor.

## Pseudosalivary swellings

A number of conditions may mimic salivary gland swelling (Table 4.1). The most common cause is probably swelling of the lymph nodes within a gland. If the

TABLE 4.1 Causes of pseudosalivary swellings

- Hypertrophy of the masseter
- Dental/mandibular lesions
- Disease of intragland lymph nodes
- Parapharyngeal space lesions

nodes drain an area of infection, reactive changes, or even lymphadenitis may occur, giving a swollen painful gland. Dental abscesses and lesions, including tumours of the mandible, may present with pseudo-salivary swellings and pain.

## SURGERY OF THE SALIVARY GLANDS

Patients with salivary gland swellings are frequently presented in surgical exams at all levels. The student will often be expected to be able to give an account of the likely diagnoses and appropriate investigations. It is unlikely that you will be expected to give a full account of an operation. However, you should at least know where the incisions are likely to be placed (Figure 4.6). The student must appreciate that the facial nerve traverses the parotid gland and as such is at risk in parotid surgery. The surgeon must have a good knowledge of the anatomy of the facial nerve (Table 4.2) in order to prevent accidental

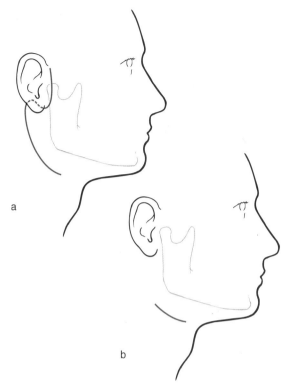

a

b

FIGURE 4.6 Points of incision for surgery to the salivary glands. (a) Incision for parotid surgery; (b) incision for submandibular gland surgery.

trauma to the nerve and the complication of facial palsy.

Other complications which may occur following parotid surgery include haematoma, salivary fistula and, rarely, Frey's syndrome. This is an unusual but interest-

TABLE 4.2 Surgical pointers to the position of the facial nerve

- The stylomastoid foramen lies at the root of the tympanomastoid suture.
- The nerve lies approximately 1-cm deep and 1-cm inferior to the cartilaginous tragal pointer.
- The nerve bisects the angle made between the mastoid process and the posterior belly of the digastric muscle.

ing condition in which the severed postsynaptic secretormotor nerve fibres which normally supply the parotid gland become abnormally redirected and regrow to innervate the sweat glands of the skin. As a result, the patient complains of sweating from the skin overlying the parotid bed during eating (Figure 4.7).

Incisions for submandibular gland surgery must be made two fingers' breadth below the ramus of the mandible in order that the marginal mandibular nerve is not severed (Figure 4.6b).

## KEY POINTS
### Salivary Gland Disease

- If more than one gland is involved in the disease process, consider a systemic condition
- When there is a uniform swelling of a gland, consider a sialadenitis/sialolithiasis
- When a lump presents within a gland, consider a tumour
- The vast majority of parotid lumps represent benign pleomorphic adenomas
- Most minor salivary gland tumours are malignant

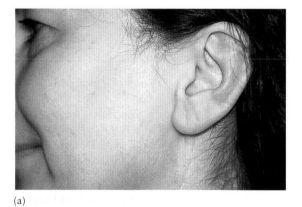

(a)

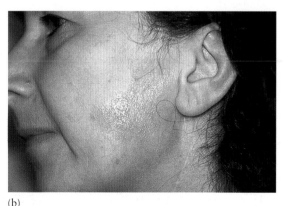

(b)

FIGURE 4.7 Frey's Syndrome: (a) before food; (b) immediately after food – notice the facial erythema and sweating. Note also the excellent healing and scar following parotid surgery.

# 5

# The larynx

Structure and function of the larynx 40

Infective and inflammatory conditions of the larynx 44

Neoplasms of the larynx 46

Hoarseness 51

Stridor 56

Emergency airway procedures 57

# STRUCTURE AND FUNCTION OF THE LARYNX

The main function of the larynx is to act as a sphincter to protect the lower airways from contamination by foods, liquids and secretions. It also allows the production of an effective cough which is essential in clearing unwanted matter from the airway. In man, it has also evolved as a highly complex organ for the production of sound vibrations. Sounds produced may then be modified by the pharynx, oral cavity, tongue, lips and teeth. Collectively, these are known as the vocal tract (Figure 5.1).

The larynx is essentially a tube which is made up of a series of cartilages and bone which are held together by interconnecting membranes, ligaments and muscles (Figures 5.2 and 5.3; see also Figure 5.8, page 43). Superiorly, the tube connects with the pharynx and thence the oral cavity, which is the shared pathway for air and food. Below the larynx, the tube becomes the trachea. Behind the larynx is the opening of the oesophagus. Food and drink are guided from the mouth to the oesophagus whilst air passes through the larynx to the trachea and lungs. These differing pathways are possible because of the structure and dynamic nature of the larynx. During swallowing, the food bolus is propelled backwards over the tongue; from here it passes in two channels called the pyriform fossa

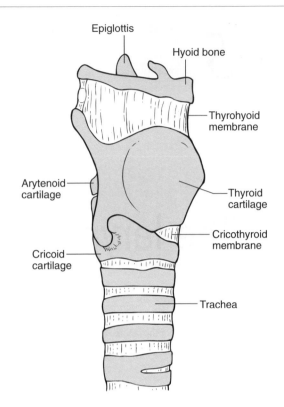

FIGURE 5.2 The external view of the larynx.

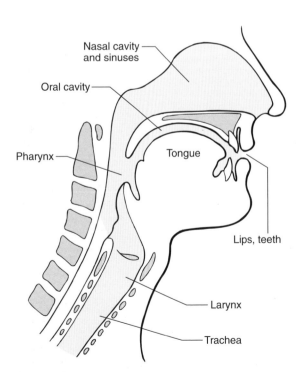

FIGURE 5.1 The vocal tract.

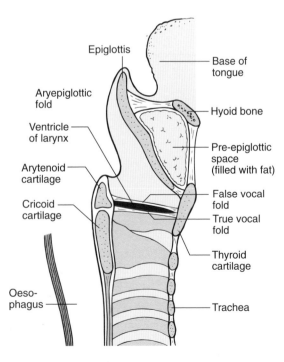

FIGURE 5.3 The internal view of the larynx.

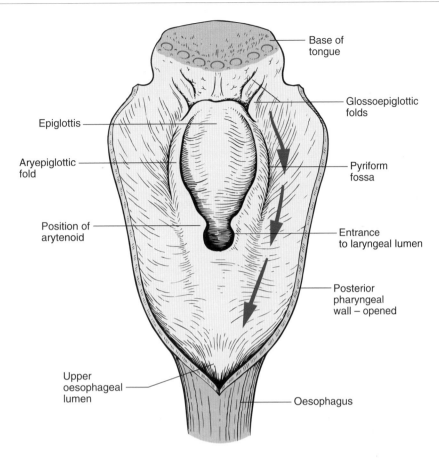

FIGURE 5.4 The relationship of the pyriform fossae (posterior view). Adapted from McMinn (1990) *Last's Anatomy*, Figure 6.29, p. 490, by permission of the publisher Churchill Livingstone.

(Figure 5.4) or pyriform sinus. These are grooves which run downwards and backwards around the laryngeal inlet and lead into the oesophagus. Swallowing is, however, a dynamic process during which the larynx is drawn upwards. This has the function of tilting the laryngeal inlet and bringing it closer to the tongue base and epiglottis, which acts a little bit like a lid.

The vocal folds (Figure 5.5) or cords, which are also sometimes called the glottis, are supported by the cartilaginous framework of the larynx. They lie suspended in the airway, being attached in front to the thyroid cartilage and behind to two small cartilages called the arytenoids which rest on the cricoid cartilage. The arytenoids can slide away from, and towards, each other and also backwards and forwards. Thus, both the position of the vocal folds, their tension and therefore the pitch of the resulting sounds, may be adjusted. The vocal folds have a complex layered structure (Figure 5.6) which allows the superficial coverings of the cords to be relatively mobile whilst the body of the cord remains stiffer. The movement of air upwards between the vocal folds causes the cover-

ings of the vocal fold to be drawn together. For a fraction of a second they meet one another until pressure builds up below the cords and they are blown apart. The resulting movements of the coverings are known as the mucosal wave (Figure 5.7). This mechanism, and defects in it, may be observed by the use of a stroboscope. This vibration of the vocal folds causes the column of air above the vocal folds to oscillate and hence sound is produced.

The glottis divides the larynx into two, the supraglottis and the subglottis (Figure 5.8). The sensation of the supraglottis is carried by the internal branch of the superior laryngeal nerve. The external branch carries motor fibres to the cricothyroid muscle. It is concerned with adjusting the tension of the vocal folds, and is the only 'laryngeal' muscle on the 'outside' of the larynx. The recurrent laryngeal nerves carry sensation to the subglottis and supply all the other laryngeal muscles. The recurrent laryngeal nerves are branches of the vagus and due to their embryological development, have a long course especially on the left side. Because of this, they are prone to injury in the neck or chest. There are several laryngeal muscles. They are all

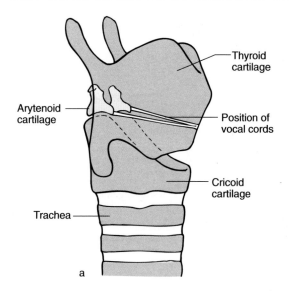

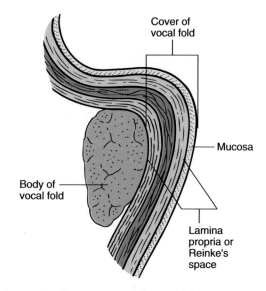

FIGURE 5.6 Micro-anatomy of the vocal fold.

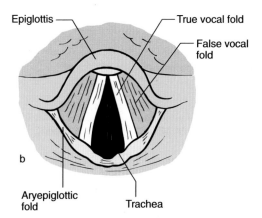

FIGURE 5.5 (a) The position of the vocal folds within the larynx. (b) View of the larynx from above.

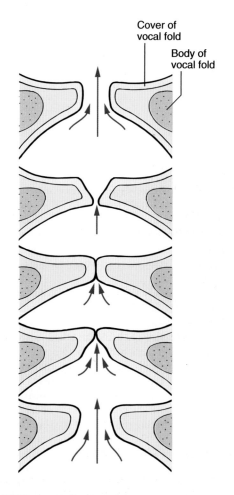

involved with adjustments of cord position and tension. Their exact individual functions are still rather poorly understood and further discussion is beyond the scope of this book. A fact much loved by examiners, however, is that the posterior crico-arytenoid muscle is the only muscle which moves the cords apart, i.e. **ab**duction, and is therefore often described as the most important muscle in the body since without its action the cords come together and no air can flow.

An important clinical point is that the glottis is the watershed for the lymph drainage of the larynx (Figure 5.8), i.e. the supraglottis drains to nodes in the

FIGURE 5.7 The mucosal wave.

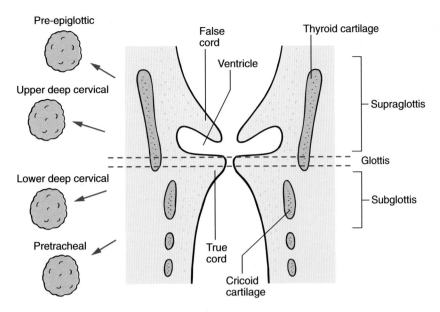

FIGURE 5.8 Anatomy and lymph drainage of the larynx.

neck. The subglottis, however, drains to the paratracheal nodes as well. The vocal folds themselves have virtually no lymph drainage. Therefore, small glottic cancers have a relatively good prognosis but sub-, supra- or transglottic tumours have a much poorer outlook.

larynx present with either voice or airway problems and not infrequently a combination of both. In children, the size of the airways is relatively and absolutely smaller. Also, the mucosa is less tightly bound down and hence may swell dramatically. The cartilaginous support for the airway is soft, and hence more prone

> **KEY POINTS**
> ## Anatomy of the Larynx
>
> - The prime function of the larynx is to protect the airway
> - The recurrent laryngeal nerves supply the muscles of the vocal folds
> - The recurrent laryngeal nerve has a long course, especially on the left side, and therefore it is susceptible to disease and trauma
> - The lymph drainage of the vocal fold is poor, therefore early glottic cancers have a good prognosis, if treated early
> - The vocal fold has a delicate layered structure and therefore surgical trauma must be kept to a minimum

> **KEY POINTS**
> ## The Child's Airway
>
> Is more at risk because:
>
> - It is smaller than in an adult
> - It is proportionately smaller than in an adult
> - The cartilaginous support is less firm, and therefore more likely to collapse
> - The mucosa is able to swell dramatically

## Diseases of the larynx

Any disease process affecting the larynx may interfere with the function of this organ. Thus diseases of the

to collapse, especially during inspiration (as in laryngomalacia). These factors make the paediatric airway more critical than the adult, and explain the relative frequency of airway problems in childhood. Laryngeal dysfunction may also lead to aspiration of saliva or liquids into the lower airways. Very occasionally, laryngeal problems may lead to 'silent' aspiration and in these circumstances the patient may present with a chest infection or pyrexia of unknown origin.

## OVERVIEW
### Diseases of the Larynx

**Congenital**
- **Laryngomalacia**
- Laryngeal web
- Subglottic stenosis
- Laryngeal cleft
- Vocal cord palsy

**Acquired**

**Trauma**
- Blunt trauma: fracture of the laryngeal skeleton
- Penetrating trauma
- Burns: chemical, heat/smoke
- **Cigarettes, alcohol fumes**

**Voice abuse**
- **Singer's nodules**
- **Reinke's oedema**
- **Vocal polyp**
- Contact ulcers

**Infections**
- **Laryngitis**
- **Epiglottitis**
- **Croup**
- Diphtheria
- Tuberculosis
- Syphilis

**Neoplastic**
- **Papillomatosis**
- **Squamous carcinoma**

**Hamartoma**
- Haemangioma

**Degenerative**
- Laryngocoele
- Vocal cord fixation

**Non-organic**
- **Functional dysphonia**

**Neurological**
- **Recurrent laryngeal nerve palsy**
- Bulbar palsy
- Motor neurone disease

# INFECTIVE AND INFLAMMATORY CONDITIONS OF THE LARYNX

## Acute laryngitis

The larynx may become inflamed in isolation or as part of a general infective process affecting the whole respiratory tract. When only the larynx is affected, it may be due to vocal abuse or voice strain as well as to exposure to irritant substances such as cigarette smoke or alcohol fumes. A hoarse voice is the most common presenting complaint and on occasions there may be complete loss of voice (aphonia). The patient may also complain of pain on speaking and swallowing. If there is an infective component, as with a generalized upper respiratory tract infection, then general malaise and slight pyrexia may be accompanying features. The diagnosis can often be made from the history and general examination of the patient. The vocal cords appear reddened and oedematous and, in fact, often the whole larynx is generally inflamed with swelling of the arytenoids and false cords, and the epiglottis may appear red at its tip. Movements of the cords are restricted but symmetrical; there is no paralysis.

Treatment in simple acute laryngitis is largely supportive consisting of voice rest, simple analgesia, steam inhalations and gentle warmth applied to the anterior neck. If cough is a feature, linctus or cough suppressants may be soothing. The importance of voice rest must be stressed to the patient since forced vocalization of an already inflamed larynx can lead to haemorrhage into the vocal fold and the resulting fibrous reaction can lead to permanent vocal disorders.

Voice rest consists of avoiding speaking when possible and if the patient has to communicate verbally, then only for a short period of time. Even then, the patient should speak in a quiet conversational voice; whispering must also be discouraged.

## Epiglottitis

This is an acute and life-threatening condition. It must always be considered as a possible diagnosis in pyrexial children with a sore throat. It is particularly hazardous because it may start with features the same as any other upper respiratory tract infection, but can rapidly progress to total airway obstruction within hours of onset. If the diagnosis is suspected then the patient, who is most commonly a child, must be admitted at once. One must also be aware that an equally dangerous variant of this condition can occur in adults. But here the inflammation tends to affect the whole of the supraglottis (supraglottitis).

The suggestive features of epiglottitis are difficulty in swallowing. This will, in time, lead to drooling of saliva and will be accompanied by a change in the voice (described as the 'hot potato voice') or change in the child's cry. This is due to a dramatic swelling of all the tissues of the supraglottis including the epiglottis. The child will be sitting up, often with arms resting on the knees and using accessory muscles of respiration. Avoid the temptation to lie the patient down since this can precipitate airway obstruction. In the same way **no** intra-oral examination should be performed unless facilities for intubation or emergency tracheostomy are available, since this again can cause a respiratory arrest. The mechanism for this is said to be due to the inflamed epiglottis falling into the airway. An alternative explanation suggests that the larynx becomes obstructed as a result of inhalation of the thick pooled secretions which fill the pharynx. This occurs when the distressed child takes a breath to cry. Whichever of these mechanisms is responsible, the important point to grasp is that the child should be kept calm, sitting up and not sent out of the Accident and Emergency department or left alone.

In the past, a lateral soft-tissue X-ray of the neck has been advocated but this is now *contraindicated* since it delays treatment and is often not diagnostic, and most importantly, it removes the patient from the resuscitation area. Some patients have died during this investigation! The agent responsible for epiglottitis is *Haemophilus influenzae* and the condition usually responds quickly to intravenous antibiotics. Once the diagnosis is suspected, the patient must be transported rapidly to the anaesthetic room in theatre where, with the most experienced anaesthetist and ENT surgeon available, the child's larynx is examined to make the diagnosis. The airway is then secured by endotracheal intubation and the child is given ventilatory support until recovery.

> ## KEY POINTS
> ### Epiglottitis
>
> - Affects children
> - Admit the patient
> - Sit the patient up
> - Do not attempt to examine the mouth
> - No X-rays
> - Get expert help early
> - Suspect the diagnosis

## Croup/acute laryngotracheobronchitis

This condition is usually viral in origin but can also be caused by *H. influenzae*, as in epiglottitis. However, here it causes a diffuse inflammation of the airways, not just the supraglottis. It tends to have a slightly longer course than epiglottitis but can be extremely serious and even life-threatening. Often the child has had a low-grade upper respiratory tract infection. There follows a rise in temperature and stridor develops; this is associated with a generalized deterioration and the child soon becomes toxic. The child is treated with intravenous antibiotics and nebulized adrenaline may be needed in severe cases. The possibility of airway obstruction must always be borne in mind and high-quality nursing and continual monitoring are essential. A period of ventilation may be necessary in some cases in which case endotracheal intubation or temporary tracheostomy may be required.

## Laryngeal diphtheria

This is included since, although nowadays it is extremely rare in the UK, it is important to bear in mind as a differential diagnosis since early recognition and treatment with antitoxin and high-dose penicillin or erythromycin is essential. The symptoms are a hoarse voice, cough and later stridor which may progress to total airway obstruction. It may often also affect the oral cavity and pharynx with membrane formation, erythema and swelling of the fauces. Exotoxin damage to the myocardium or peripheral nerves can occur. If there is any doubt in the diagnosis, take a swab and treat as diphtheria until proven otherwise.

## Chronic laryngitis

Chronic inflammation of the larynx is often multifactorial. The most important single aetiological factor is cigarette smoke. Often the patient can trace the symptoms to a nasty upper respiratory tract infection, after which they have been hoarse. Once inflammation has occurred it is sustained due to a combination of factors such as vocal abuse, chronic bronchitis, sinusitis leading to a purulent postnasal drip, environmental pollutants, acid reflux and alcohol fumes (Figure 5.9). Rarer causes include tuberculosis, leprosy, syphilis, scleroma and fungal infections, and here vocal cord biopsy may be required in order to establish the diagnosis.

The patient complains of a hoarse voice and examination of the larynx will often show erythematous vocal cords which may be thickened and oedematous. The vocal folds have a very poor lymph drainage and as a result even a small amount of oedema in the submucosal lamina propria or Reinke's space will at best be very slow to resolve and in some cases may become permanent (Reinke's oedema). Chronic inflammation

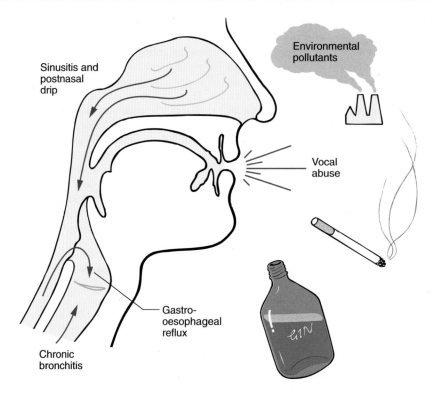

Sinusitis and postnasal drip

Environmental pollutants

Vocal abuse

Gastro-oesophageal reflux

Chronic bronchitis

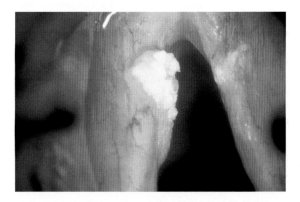

FIGURE 5.9 Causes of chronic laryngitis.

of the laryngeal mucosa may lead to dysplasia or carcinoma *in situ* and these patients must be watched carefully for the development of invasive carcinoma.

Management of chronic laryngitis consists of intensive speech therapy and removal of the causative factors. The role of surgery in chronic laryngitis is largely diagnostic nowadays, and stripping the mucosa of the vocal folds which was once so frequently performed, has now been recognized as destroying its vital layered structure. As a result, this has largely been abandoned except where micro-invasive malignancy is suspected. In patients where oedema persists in the vocal fold (Reinke's oedema), some specialists would incise the mucosa and suck out the underlying oedematous fluid, thus hoping to preserve the layered nature of the cord.

FIGURE 5.10 A small squamous cell carcinoma limited to the left vocal cord (T1a). Published with the kind permission of Mr G. Bates FRCS.

## NEOPLASMS OF THE LARYNX

### Malignant tumours of the larynx

By far the most common malignant tumour of the larynx is squamous cell carcinoma (Figure 5.10). Here the most important aetiological factor is cigarette smoking. The greater the number of cigarettes smoked per day and the longer the patient has smoked, the greater the relative risk. When combined with heavy alcohol intake, the risk is greater still. It is important to realise that the larynx includes more than just the vocal folds; in fact, the larynx can be divided into supraglottic, glottic and subglottic regions. Each region comprises a number of sites:

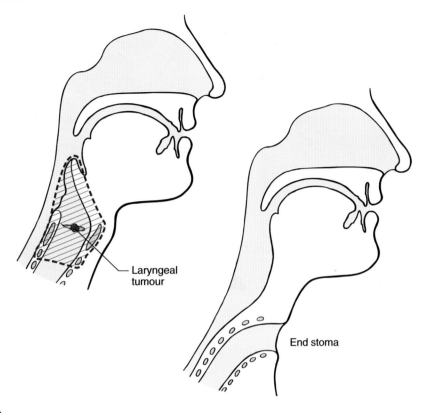

FIGURE 5.11 Total laryngectomy.

- Supraglottis    Epiglottis, false cords, ventricles, arytenoids, aryepiglottic folds
- Glottis    Vocal folds (including the anterior and posterior commisures which are the gaps between the vocal folds, front and back)
- Subglottis    Inferior surface of the vocal folds and also the trachea

## Staging of laryngeal cancer

Much of the following discussion refers equally to the staging of other head and neck cancers. The concept behind staging is that, by laying down internationally accepted criteria by which tumours may be assessed, those professionals involved in the treatment of such cases can, with some degree of unity, decide upon treatment strategies for their patients. Furthermore, the results of treatments for each stage can be compared accurately between different medical centres and for differing treatment regimens.

Understanding the anatomical areas described above is most important when staging tumours of the larynx via the TNM classification. It is not necessary for the student to memorize such classifications.

Indeed many ENT surgeons would not be able to recall it accurately, it is far better to look up the current classification and avoid mistakes.

## Symptoms of laryngeal cancer

The primary symptom of carcinoma of the vocal cords is hoarseness. Since a small lesion affecting the vocal folds will cause symptoms early, and due to the poor lymph drainage of the true cords, cancers at this site tend to have a good prognosis (the five-year survival is 95%). It is important that any patient who has a persistent hoarse voice for more than three weeks is referred to the ENT department as a matter of urgency to exclude such a tumour. Cancers which arise in other regions of the larynx, namely the sub- and supraglottic regions, unfortunately do not have such definite and early symptoms. They may cause irritation in the throat, cough, referred otalgia or may present with a node in the neck. It is not until late that airway compromise or hoarseness develops. As a general rule, any patient who presents with an unexplained node in the neck must be referred to the ENT department for examination of the likely primary sites of such tumours, i.e. endoscopic examination of the whole aerodigestive tract.

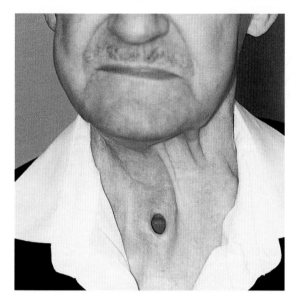

FIGURE 5.12 A laryngectomy patient.

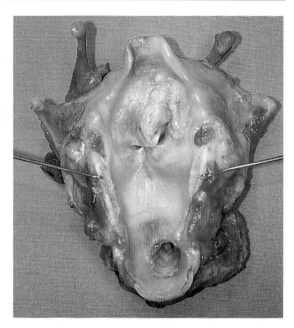

FIGURE 5.13 An operative laryngectomy specimen. The larynx has been opened from behind. Note the left-sided carcinoma affecting the vocal cord and supraglottis.

## Treatment options for laryngeal cancer

The primary treatment options for laryngeal cancers are:

- Endoscopic removal
- Radiotherapy
- Radical surgical excision

On many occasions, treatment will be a planned combination of surgery and radiotherapy. Generally speaking, small tumours may either be treated with primary radiotherapy or local, often endoscopic, excision. The advantage of radiotherapy in these cases is that the voice is preserved intact. Unless the lesion is extremely small, surgical excision generally has a more deleterious effect upon the voice. It is, however, quick and without the other complications of radiotherapy such as mucositis, skin reactions and troublesome dry throat. The decision as to which treatment option should be employed will depend not least upon the patient's informed choice.

Small- and medium-sized tumours, i.e. T1, T2 and some T3 will usually be treated with radiotherapy and 'salvage surgery'. That is to say, that the primary treatment is radiotherapy and should the tumour recur, the patient may be offered radical surgical excision. Large tumours (T3 and T4) are most often treated with radical surgery primarily and planned combined radiotherapy which may be administered pre- or postoperatively. Total laryngectomy (Figures 5.11 to 5.13) is an effective and well-trusted operation for treatment of advanced laryngeal cancer. It is, however, mutilating, demands a permanent stoma in the neck

and reduces the patient's communicating ability to oesophageal speech at best (see below). Over the years, innovative surgeons have devised more conservative operations in which some part of the uninvolved larynx can be preserved, with the intent that voice restoration can be improved. Such operations include hemilaryngectomy, either vertical or horizontal, and near total laryngectomy.

Chemotherapy has little part to play in curative treatment but can be useful in palliation. Some advances have been made in recent years in the area of photodynamic therapy but as yet this has not reached the clinical forum. Recently, much interest has been focused on gene markers for laryngeal cancers, for example the *p53* gene which it is hoped will be helpful in identifying those individuals at risk of developing such disease and also in helping to determine individual long-term prognosis for laryngeal cancer patients.

## The multidisciplinary approach

The treatment of laryngeal cancers, as with other cancers of the head and neck, is best concentrated in dedicated regional cancer units. Here the multidisciplinary team is paramount and this should ideally include a specialist histopathologist, radiologist, radiotherapist, ENT surgeon, oral/maxillofacial surgeon, plastic and reconstructive surgeon, specialist

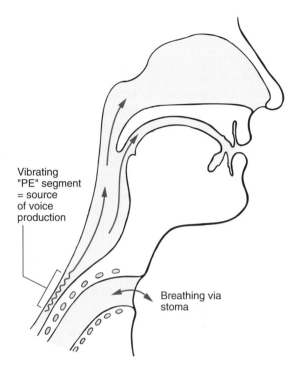

FIGURE 5.14 Oesophageal speech in laryngectomy patient.

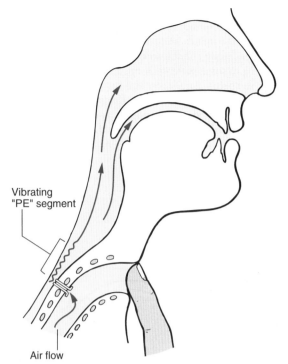

FIGURE 5.15 Voice production with a tracheo-oesophageal fistula after laryngectomy.

trained nurses, speech therapist, physiotherapist, dietician, Macmillan nurse and community support team. Each of these members of the team is essential to the overall care and welfare of the patient. Therefore, treatment of head and neck cancer patients is not simply a case of surgery or radiotherapy.

## Voice restoration after laryngectomy

The importance of patient motivation and an interested speech therapist cannot be overemphasized in the successful acquisition of speech after laryngectomy. Oesophageal speech (Figure 5.14) offers the prospect of near normal verbal communication in those patients who can acquire it. The basic principle is that air is swallowed into the stomach and then regurgitated into the oesophagus. The soft tissues in this area are forced to vibrate as a result and hence sound is produced. This sound may then be modified by the mouth and tongue to form articulate speech. The main problem with this form of speech is that it is rather gruff and is not well suited to the female voice. Also, only a small amount of air can be swallowed at a time and hence speech tends to take on a rather staccato quality. The latter problem can be much improved by the surgical formation of a tracheo-oesophageal fistula, which may be created at the time of the initial surgery, or at some later date. Into this is fitted a one-way valve

(Figures 5.15 and 5.16). This allows air to be forced from the lungs through the valve into the vibrating segment of the oesophagus (the pharyngo-oesophageal segment) when the patient occludes his tracheostome with his thumb. This has the advantage of increasing fluency and strength of voice. In those patients who are unable to achieve such speech, mechanical vibrating devices (Figure 5.17) may be used to produce the

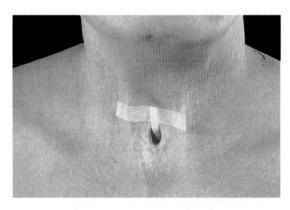

FIGURE 5.16 A laryngectomy patient with a Blom–Singer valve taped in place. Published with kind permission of Mr G. Bates FRCS.

sound source. The device is held against the neck and the resulting sound vibration is modified by movements of the mouth and tongue to form speech. It is, however, rather robotic-sounding speech which is not pleasing to some patients. It must be remembered that prior to speech acquisition and for those unfortunate patients who never develop effective speech, much psychological and social support is essential if complete social isolation is to be avoided.

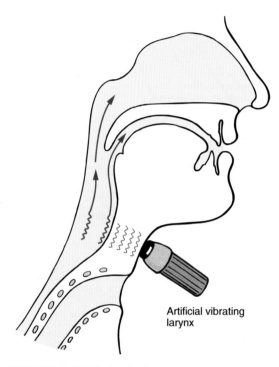

Artificial vibrating larynx

FIGURE 5.17 Artificial vibrating larynx.

## KEY POINTS
### Laryngeal Cancer

- Is caused by smoking
- Early glottic cancer has a good prognosis
- Hoarseness is a consistent and early sign when the vocal cord is affected
- Accurate staging and assessment is vital
- Patients should be assessed in a multidisciplinary combined clinic
- Treatment may be surgical, radiotherapy, or a combination of both
- Effective speech is achieved by the majority of patients after laryngectomy

## CASE STUDY

Walter, a 77-year-old ex-serviceman, and smoker of 15 cigarettes a day for most of his adult life, presents to his GP complaining of a hoarse voice for the last six weeks. He also admits to some left-sided earache, particularly on swallowing. He lives alone since the death of his wife six years ago, and has lost touch with his family. He is known to the practice since he has had a problem with alcohol abuse in recent years. Indirect laryngoscopy shows a mass arising from the left vocal cord, which is not mobile. The neck, chest and abdomen are normal.

1  What is the most likely diagnosis?
2  How should the patient be investigated?
3  List the other agencies/specialities which should be involved with this case.

**Comments**

1  Squamous cell carcinoma of the larynx must be considered in any patient who has a hoarse voice for more than three weeks. In this case the patients smoking history and referred otalgia are highly suggestive of this diagnosis.

2  The patient must have a microlaryngoscopy and biopsy of the abnormal vocal cord. In addition full pan-endoscopy should be performed in order to exclude a second, smoking induced primary tumour. A pre-operative chest X-ray should be performed in order to exclude a carcinoma of the lung. It is important to examine the neck in order to pick up any metastatic tumour deposits.

3  In addition to the GP and an ENT surgeon, the head and neck team should include an oncologist/radiotherapist, speech therapist, dietician, head and neck community liaison nurse/Macmillan nurse, social worker and possibly an alcohol dependence worker.

## Benign tumours of the larynx

Papillomata of the larynx are the least rare of these tumours and are discussed further below. Remember that any of the constituent tissues of the larynx may undergo neoplastic transformation, for example chondromata, fibromata and haemangiomata may all occur. They may affect both children and adults, and present with the usual laryngeal symptoms of hoarseness and airway compromise.

## Laryngeal papillomatosis

This is a condition most often seen in children and juveniles but it can also appear in adulthood. The underlying cause is infection with the human papilloma virus (HPV).

The route of transmission is probably inhalation. However, why some individuals are affected and others are not is not fully understood. It seems likely that a defect in some part of the immune system is responsible. The extent of the disease process is variable and may affect only a small part of the larynx, or may be widespread, involving the whole of the respiratory tree, including the trachea and rarely the bronchi. Those children affected can undergo spontaneous regression at any stage, most commonly at puberty. However, this is not uniformly the case. Regression in adulthood is rare. The most common site to be affected is the vocal cord and hence the symptoms consist of hoarseness. In the most severe cases, stridor may develop.

## Treatment

Surgical treatment should aim to preserve the airway and avoid causing too much scarring to the larynx since otherwise, if/when regression takes place, the patient is left at best hoarse, and at worst aphonic with an incompetent larynx. Modern treatment consists in removal of the papillomata, most often using a laser. Microlaryngoscopy is preferred in order adequately to visualize the area and so avoid excessive damage to the delicate structure of the vocal folds. Normally several removals are required over many years, since the papillomata regrow, sometimes at an alarming rate. Very occasionally, the airway is so occluded by papillomata that a tracheostomy or even a laryngectomy is required. However, even then, problems may develop due to papillomata growing at the stoma. Efforts have been made to trigger the immune system in these cases, with moderate success, using systemic steroids or interferon. Malignant transformation to squamous cell carcinomas has been described in adults and as such histological examination of any removed papillomata is mandatory.

# HOARSENESS

This is the cardinal symptom of laryngeal disease. We have already discussed many of the causes of hoarseness. However, some are still outstanding. The most important causes are summarized below:

*Inflammation*
  Acute
  Chronic
      specific
      non-specific
*Neoplastic*
  Benign
      papilloma
      haemangioma
  Malignant
      squamous carcinoma
*Neurological*
  Central
      cerebrovascular accident
      multiple sclerosis

## KEY POINTS
### Avoiding Voice Problems

- Drink plenty of liquid (not including tea, coffee, alcohol or fizzy drinks). Aim to have 8–10 drinks per day
- Get enough sleep, as being tired will affect your voice in the same way that it would affect any muscular problem
- Eat regular meals and try to eat a balanced diet
- Avoid irritants such as spicy foods, tobacco, smoky places, excessive dust and alcohol
- Keep your bedroom and lounge humidified appropriately. If you have central heating on, this will dry the atmosphere so put a bowl of water near the radiators or a damp towel on them
- Do not suck medicated lozenges unless you have a sore throat. These numb the throat, allowing you to do more damage and the menthol also has a drying effect on your vocal cords
- To keep your mouth moist suck ordinary pastilles or chew gum

**If you have an acute infection take the following steps:**
- Increase your fluid intake
- Take steam inhalations twice a day
- Rest your voice or use it as little as possible but do not whisper as this will strain your vocal cords even more!
- Do not gargle with aspirin

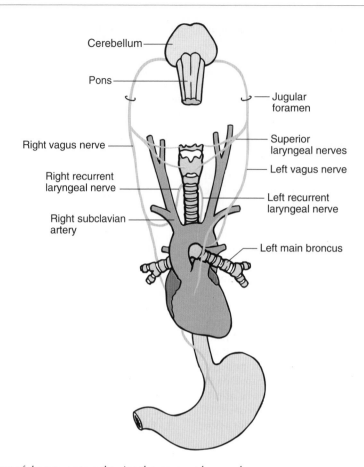

FIGURE 5.18 The course of the vagus nerve showing the recurrent laryngeal nerve.

Peripheral
    recurrent laryngeal nerve palsy
    motor neurone disease
*Mechanical*
    Singer's nodules
    Vocal polyp
    Vocal cord cysts
*Non-organic*
    Functional dysphonia

Many ENT departments now run a specialized voice clinic where patients with hoarseness and other voice problems can be assessed. Such a clinic will usually comprise an ENT surgeon/laryngologist and a speech therapist, and occasionally a voice/singing teacher. In addition, there will be specialized equipment (such as a videolaryngostroboscope) in order to examine the vocal cords and their movements.

Remember that professional voice users are not just singers and actors but anyone who uses their voice regularly at work, e.g. receptionists, secretaries, policemen, solicitors, doctors, etc.

# Neurological causes of hoarseness

When brainstem tissue is damaged as a result of some form of cerebrovascular accident, trauma or indeed tumour, the motor supply of the larynx may be affected. When this occurs, it is usually as a result of extensive and severe brain damage. In these circumstances, phonation is less important than protection of the airway. Indeed, many patients who have extensive brain injuries die of pneumonia as a result of aspiration.

## Central causes

### Recurrent laryngeal nerve palsy

The recurrent laryngeal nerve (Figure 5.18) is a branch of the vagus nerve and due to its embryological development has an unusually long course, especially on the left side. On this side, it runs around the arch of the aorta before passing upwards over the pleura and into the neck. Here it runs in a groove

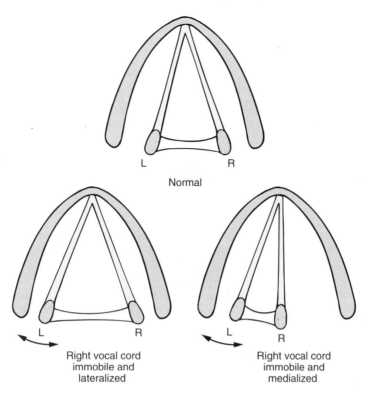

FIGURE 5.19 Positions of the vocal cords when paralysed.

between the trachea and oesophagus before finally entering the larynx. As a result of its great length, the nerve is frequently damaged in diseases of, or surgery to, any of its close relations, i.e. the lungs, oesophagus and thyroid gland, as well as being at risk in many intrathoracic operations. Prior to thyroid surgery, the vocal cord mobility should be checked to establish whether or not there is any pre-existing palsy.

In vocal cord palsy remember the 'rule of thirds'

⅓ idiopathic
⅓ surgery
⅓ neoplasia

### Investigation of vocal fold palsy

When a patient presents with a hoarse voice and the cause is an unexplained immobile vocal fold, it should be assumed that the underlying pathology is a malignancy until proven otherwise. A chest X-ray is mandatory as this may frequently show an underlying bronchial carcinoma. If no abnormality is seen on chest X-ray, a computed tomography scan from skull base to hilum of the lung is suggested, since this will demonstrate most other neoplastic lesions which can involve the recurrent laryngeal nerve. Further investi-

gation of suspicious areas may include ultrasound of the thyroid gland and rigid endoscopy of the areodigestive tract under general anaesthesia. Often the cause of the palsy is unexplained and is most frequently attributed to a postviral neuropathy.

The vocal cords may be immobile for reasons other than neurological defects however. It is important to remember that the synovial crico-arytenoid joint may become fixed, for example as a result of severe rheumatoid arthritis, or acid reflux as well as carcinoma involving the joint. In these circumstances, direct laryngoscopy, under general anaesthesia, will allow assessment of the mobility of the joint and in difficult cases electrophysiological testing can be very helpful.

The final position (Figure 5.19) that the cord adopts is important since, if it is lateral, the voice will be poor and the airway good, and vice versa, if the cord is medial, the voice will be good and the airway may be a problem. There is much written in older texts concerning the underlying pathology determining the position of the cord. This is best forgotten since at best it is unreliable and at worst misleading. With the advent of modern imaging techniques, these 'rules' should be regarded as interesting observations and no more.

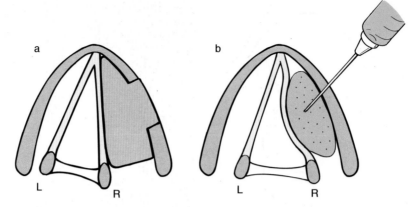

FIGURE 5.20 Vocal fold medialization procedures. (a) Right vocal fold medialized by insertion of a silastic implant (thyroplasty). (b) Right vocal fold medialized by injection of Teflon.

## Treatment

When treating vocal fold palsy, one must remember that the prime function of the larynx is to protect the lower respiratory tree, and thus one must balance voice against airway and aspiration.

In vocal fold palsy there are two basic patterns; firstly the cord which is lateralized, i.e. **ab**ducted. This situation most often occurs in unilateral vocal cord palsy, the voice is weak, as is the cough, but the airway is good. Initial treatment will be aimed at maximizing the function of the other vocal fold in an attempt to allow it to slightly cross over the midline and meet its partner. This may be achieved by speech therapy. Some 'postviral' vocal cord palsies will recover spontaneously and as a result most ENT surgeons will allow a period of recovery of at least six months prior to any surgical intervention. However, if the cause is known (e.g. a terminally ill patient with carcinoma of the lung causing a recurrent laryngeal nerve palsy), this period of observation would be inappropriate and intervention is required. The aim

of treatment in these cases is to medialize the vocal cord. This can be achieved by (Figure 5.20):

(i) injecting a thick fluid lateral to the cord and hence pushing it towards the midline; Teflon is the most commonly used substance in the UK;
(ii) laryngeal framework surgery which involves surgical manipulation of the thyroid and/or arytenoid cartilages; here, the cartilaginous framework, within which the vocal folds are suspended, is modified and hence their position altered.

In the second pattern of vocal cord palsy, the cord adopts a medial position, i.e. it is **ad**ducted. This is most often seen in bilateral cord palsies and here the airway effects are predominant over the voice, which is often good as is the cough. The surgical aim here is either to reposition the cord more laterally or to excise part of the cord (Figure 5.21) in an attempt to improve the airway. It is in this situation that aspiration may be induced and, as a result, surgery should be cautious. In cases where the airway is critical, tracheostomy (Figure 5.22) may be required.

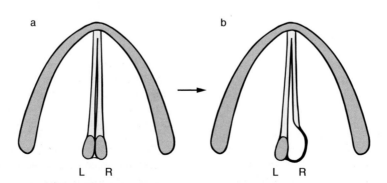

FIGURE 5.21 (a) Bilateral vocal fold palsy with airway compromise. (b) Improvement in the airway after right arytenoidectomy.

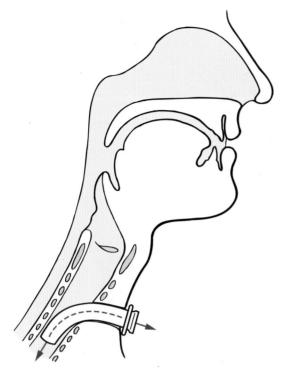

FIGURE 5.22 Air flow after tracheostomy.

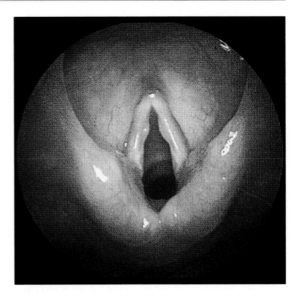

FIGURE 5.23 Singer's nodules; these occur as a result of voice abuse.

## KEY POINTS
### Vocal Cord Palsy

- A hoarse voice is the usual presenting feature
- Is often caused by bronchial cancer and this must be excluded
- Surgery may improve both the voice and the patient's cough
- Remember to balance the voice – airway – aspiration

## Mechanical causes of hoarseness

### Vocal cord nodules (Figure 5.23)

Often known as singer's or screamer's nodules, these are formed as a result of vocal abuse. They cause hoarseness and gruffness of the voice. In some professional voice users, e.g. singers, this vocal quality may be characteristic and no treatment is requested

## CASE STUDY

Victoria is 26 years old and is currently trying to break into television. She has been auditioning for the last few months on a regular basis. She is now finding that her voice, which has always had a rather husky quality, is becoming very hoarse and she is finding it difficult to perform, especially when she is asked to sing. She is very concerned that her voice may interfere with her job prospects. She smokes 10 cigarettes a day and is always 'on the go'. Examination confirms the fact that she is quite hoarse, and her vocal cords have 'swellings' bilaterally.

1. What is the most likely diagnosis?
2. What should be her first line of treatment?
3. Does surgery have a role to play in this condition?

### Comments
1. She has singer's or screamer's nodules.
2. In the majority of cases the nodules will resolve with a course of speech therapy.
3. In those cases which fail to resolve after speech therapy, surgery may be required in order remove the nodules, taking care to cause as little disruption as possible to the coverings of the vocal fold in order to preserve the mucosal wave.

or required. More often, however, the patient dislikes their gruff voice and examination of the larynx will show small, usually white, nodular thickenings of the vocal folds bilaterally. These form at the area of maximal forceful glottic closure, i.e. the junction of the anterior third and posterior two-thirds of the cords. Initially, they are soft and probably result from a small haemorrhage into the vocal cord. With time, fibrosis occurs and the nodules become firm. Treatment consists of speech therapy which is often successful, especially in the soft variety. If the nodules are resistant to conservative management, then surgical excision may be required.

## Vocal cord polyps and cysts

Once again, these lesions will present with a hoarse voice. Inflammation of the vocal cord from whichever of the causes already mentioned will lead to oedema in Reinke's space or lamina propria. When the whole length of the cord is oedematous, the condition is known as Reinke's oedema.

When the inflammation is localized to one region of the cord, cysts or polyps may develop. A vocal cord cyst forms when the oedema localizes under the coverings of the cord and remains contained within it. A vocal polyp (Figure 5.24) results from oedema more superficially in the cord which then prolapses into the airway. Small cysts may be difficult to recognize without the aid of stroboscopic examination of the altered mucosal wave. Vocal cord polyps can also be missed without careful examination since, when large, they may hang from a thin pedicle and on inspiration may 'hide' under the vocal fold and only on expiration are they forced up into the airway to be recognized. Removal is necessary to submit the lesion to histological examination.

## Functional dysphonia

Previously known as 'hysterical dysphonia' this is a diagnosis which actually includes a wide variety of non-organic voice problems and a fuller discussion of these is not appropriate here. The patient may present with a hoarse or weak voice which tires easily, a high or abnormally pitched voice, or even no voice at all. These problems may be attributed to laryngeal dysfunction resulting from vocal strain, stress and psychological or psychiatric problems. The patient may have experienced some form of stress or major life event at the time of the onset of their symptoms. Not infrequently, a friend or relation may have recently developed some serious throat problem. Treatment of these patients involves

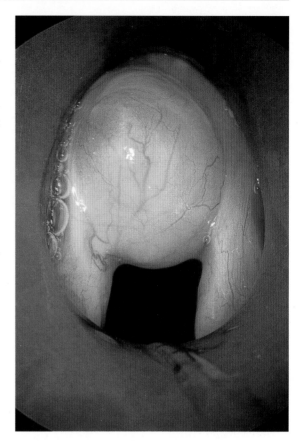

FIGURE 5.24 A large vocal cord polyp.

explanation of the problem, firm reassurance that there is no serious cause. Speech therapy will relieve laryngeal tension and retrain the patient in good vocal habits. On rare occasions, the help of a psychiatrist may be required.

## STRIDOR

Stridor is noisy breathing. The noise which is produced varies in quality depending which part of the airway is responsible for its production. Laryngeal stridor has a high-pitched musical quality and is produced on inspiration. Those noises which are produced from the oropharynx are called 'stertor' or 'snoring'. Stridor is more common in children due to the differing anatomical and physiological features of the paediatric larynx which can predispose to airway obstruction (see page 43).

It is important to realize that the resistance to air flow though a tube, and hence the work of breathing, is inversely related to the square of the tube's diameter. This means that a small narrowing in the airway will dramatically increase the effort required to breath.

The causes of stridor are summarised below:

*Congenital*
- Laryngomalacia (an excessively 'floppy' airway with a tendency to collapse on inspiration)
- Vocal cord web
- Vocal cord palsy
- Subglottic stenosis

*Acquired*
Acute
- Trauma, e.g. fractured larynx
- Foreign body
- Angioneurotic oedema, i.e. allergic reaction
- Epiglottitis
- Croup
- Vocal cord palsy, e.g. iatrogenic

Chronic
- Vocal cord palsy
- Carcinoma
- Subglottic stenosis, e.g. after prolonged intubation
- Papillomata
- Vocal cord polyp/cyst
- External compression, e.g. thyroid mass

## Management of stridor

In the acute situation, even a rapidly taken history will usually give the diagnosis. However, differentiating between croup and epiglottitis can be difficult. Features which are suggestive of epiglottitis are:

- Shorter history (12–18 hours)
- High temperature (≥38°C)
- Drooling
- No cough
- Prominent dysphagia

These signs and symptoms are, however, only suggestive and in either case the child should be admitted. Formal assessment of the child's airway should be undertaken by an experienced team and where necessary endotracheal intubation and ventilation should be used. If any doubt remains, cover with antibiotics and consider intravenous steroids, nebulized adrenaline and humidification. The prime concern in all patients with acute stridor is to maintain a secure airway. It is far safer to intervene to secure the airway early, rather than to try to follow a conservative course.

# EMERGENCY AIRWAY PROCEDURES

## Assessment of the critical airway

Simply looking and listening to the patient will give you a lot of information about their airway. Emergency situations can be frightening for all concerned, but try not to panic, think in logical patterns and appear confident and try to reassure the patient who will undoubtedly be far more frightened than you!

## Try to answer the following questions:

- Does the patient require admission to hospital?
- Will admission and observation suffice or is the clinical picture deteriorating such that active intervention will be required?
- If intervention is required do you have time to call an expert or do you need to do something *now*? If so, consider oxygen with or without antibiotics, nebulized adrenaline, intubate, laryngotomy, tracheostomy.

## Start by looking at the patient:

- What is their colour ? Are they blue ?
- Look for intercostal recession/tracheal tug.
- What is their respiratory rate?

## Then listen to the patient:

- Are they able to talk in sentences/in short phrases/words only/not at all?
- Do they have inspiratory stridor (laryngeal) or expiratory wheeze (tracheo-bronchial)?
- What is the history?

## Look at the observations chart and other investigations:

- Respiratory rate. Climbing?
- Pyrexial?
- Oxygen saturation. Falling?
- Pulsus paradoxicus? This is the difference between pulse pressure (systolic versus diastolic) in inspiration and the pulse pressure in expiration. Normal is < 10 mmHg.

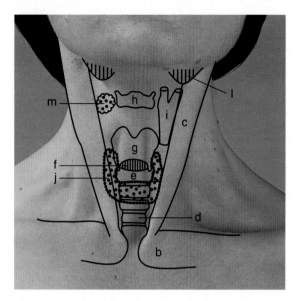

FIGURE 5.25 Surface anatomy of the neck: (b) heads of clavicles; (c) sternomastoid; (d) trachea; (e) cricoid cartilage; (f) cricothyroid membrane; (g) thyroid cartilage; (h) hyoid bone; (i) carotid artery; (j) thyroid gland; (l) submandibular gland; (m) jugulodigastric lymph node.

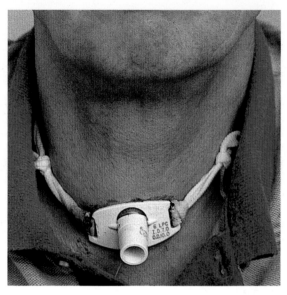

FIGURE 5.26 A tracheostomy.

## Endotracheal intubation

This is the first-line treatment for acute airway obstruction where experienced staff are available and adequate equipment is at hand. All casualty departments and hospital wards will have an endotracheal intubation (ET) tube on the resuscitation trolley. Placement of an ET tube is a skill that all anaesthetists and casualty doctors attain and practise regularly. All medical staff should at some point in their training be instructed in intubation. The introduction of the laryngeal mask airway, which is somewhat easier to insert, may become more popular in the future. However, it does not protect the airway from blood, saliva or vomit as effectively as a cuffed ET tube. On occasions, endotracheal intubation may not be possible due to poor access, inadequate equipment or unskilled staff. In this situation, other manoeuvres are needed to establish an airway. Which of the following methods are used will depend on the training and experience of the staff in attendance as well as the equipment available.

## Laryngotomy

Here, a hollow tube is introduced into the lumen of the larynx via a percutaneous route. The easiest and most commonly available instrument, at least in the hospital setting, is a wide-bore intravenous cannula. This is inserted into the neck in the midline through the cricothyroid membrane (Figure 5.25). Its position can be confirmed by withdrawing air into a fluid filled syringe; bubbles will be seen. Once in position it should be secured with tape and oxygen supply attached. Two or three such needles can be inserted if necessary. Custom-made, specially designed kits are available for use in this procedure and are often available in casualty. However, in desperation, all manner of tubes have been inserted through the cricothyroid membrane and saved lives as a result; for example, a steak knife to make the incision and a hollow barrel of a Biro pen to maintain the airway.

## Tracheostomy (Figures 5.22 and 5.26)

Here, a hole is made in the front wall of the trachea and a tube maintains this airway. Most commonly, this is performed as an elective procedure in patients who require long-term assisted ventilation or as part of some head and neck or airway operation. In the emergency situation, a 'crash' tracheostomy may be required. Here, the technique is modified somewhat; a scalpel blade is used to make a longitudinal incision in the neck, whilst the other hand supports the larynx in the midline and provides some pressure on the thyroid isthmus as it is divided in an attempt to minimize bleeding. The blade is plunged into the trachea and twisted side-ways to keep the incision in the trachea open. Then a tube may be inserted into the airway, which is then secured, and haemorrhage dealt with.

In recent years, 'percutaneous tracheostomy' has become popular especially amongst anaesthetists working in intensive treatment units. This technique involves passing a needle into the tracheal lumen, through which is passed a guidewire. Dilators of increasing size are passed over the wire until a tracheosotomy tube can be inserted.

## Tracheostomy tubes (Figure 5.27)

Tracheostomy tubes are used to maintain an airway in a patient who has had an artificial opening in the trachea surgically constructed. This opening, or 'stoma' is sited in the anterior neck. There are many different varieties of tube and the details of these are not important. What is important to understand is the basic principles of the common designs so that the appropriate tube may be selected for your patient.

### Inner tubes

These are tubes which fit within the lumen of the outer or main tube and are also slightly longer than it in order to project a little beyond the end of the main tube. This allows any crusts to form preferentially on the inner tube which may then be easily removed, cleaned and replaced.

### Plastic versus metal tubes

Plastic, disposable tubes are used when the tracheostomy is temporary or when a cuff is required to protect the lower respiratory tree, or when artificial ventilation is required. Metal tubes, which are usually made of inert silver are used in the long-term tracheostomized patient. There are many different types of silver tubes which vary slightly in their length and curvature.

### Cuffed versus non-cuffed tubes

A cuff is a high-volume, low-pressure balloon which may be inflated via a separate channel. This balloon, when inflated, prevents air or fluid leaking around the tube. Cuffed tubes are used if positive-pressure ventilation is required or if there is a danger of contamination of the lower airways with blood, saliva or gastric contents. All cuffed tubes are made of plastic. In all other

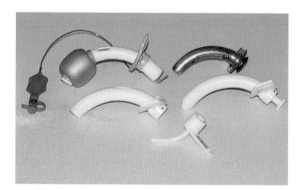

FIGURE 5.27 A variety of tracheostomy tubes.

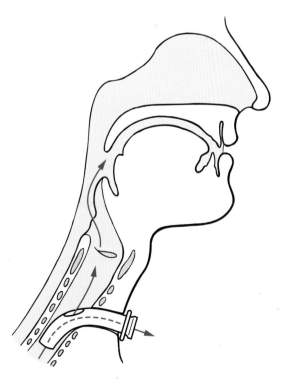

FIGURE 5.28 Airflow with a fenestrated tracheostomy tube.

situations, a non-cuffed tube is generally preferred since prolonged inflation of the cuff can lead to damage to the tracheal lining and subsequent tracheal stenosis.

### Fenestrated versus non-fenestrated tubes

A fenestration is a small hole made in the greater curvature of the tube. This hole allows air to pass upwards through the cords when the stoma is occluded by the patient's finger, and as a result, voice can be produced (Figure 5.28). This is useful in patients who have medialzed and immobile cords where air cannot be inhaled in the usual manner (hence the need for a tracheostomy). Non-fenestrated tubes are used where there is a danger of aspiration or where the position/structure of the cords does not allow the production of useful voice. A one-way speaking valve may be introduced into this system to automatically close off the tracheostomy outlet during expiration and hence produce 'hands' free' speech.

### Paediatric tubes

These are smaller and softer than the adult variety. They also have a curve and flanges for tape attachment which better fit the infant neck and trachea.

## Care of a tracheostomy

When the upper respiratory pathways are bypassed as in a tracheostomy, the humidification functions of the nose are lost. As a result, the trachea quickly becomes dry and tends to crust, and so obstruct the trachea and block the tube. Thus all patients must have humidification of the air they breath and regular suctions of the lower airways in order to prevent such problems postoperatively.

In time, the lining of the trachea changes to a more robust squamous variety and the need for humidification reduces. Patients must be shown how to clean and care for their tubes prior to their discharge home.

# 6

# The oesophagus and dysphagia

Structure and function of the oesophagus  62

Congenital oesophageal abnormalities  62

Oesophageal foreign bodies  62

Gastro-oesophageal reflux disease and hiatus hernia  64

Caustic ingestion  65

Neurological causes of dysphagia  66

Achalasia  66

Pharyngeal pouch  66

Postcricoid web  68

Oesophageal tumours  68

Investigation of dysphagia  70

# STRUCTURE AND FUNCTION OF THE OESOPHAGUS

The oesophagus is a muscular tube which connects the pharynx above to the stomach below. The oesophagus is described as starting at the level of the sixth cervical vertebra, i.e. at the level of the lower border of the cricoid cartilage. It is 25 cm long in the adult, and enters the stomach at the level of the eleventh thoracic vertebra. Its function is to propel food and liquid to the stomach. Diseases which affect the oesophagus usually present with some difficulty in swallowing. This is one of the many areas where ENT overlaps with other specialties, in this case gastrointestinal physician and cardiothoracic surgeon. It is vital that there is close liaison between each specialty in order to benefit the doctor and patient alike.

# CONGENITAL OESOPHAGEAL ABNORMALITIES

Such abnormalities of the oesophagus are rare but may account for some cases of infant death or may lead to problems with feeding or failure to thrive. Since the trachea and lungs develop from the foregut, abnormalities which involve both the respiratory tree and oesophagus are most frequent. Various types of oesophageal atresia and stenosis are found, often in combination with abnormal communications with the trachea (Figure 6.1). Occasionally, a congenital tracheo-oesophageal fistula may be present without any atresia or stenosis of the oesophagus.

Obviously, the ability of the child to survive beyond birth will depend upon the type and severity of the abnormality. In mild cases, the infant may present with choking attacks, feeding problems or chest infections whereas in severe cases the child may die at, or soon after, birth from respiratory failure. Less severe abnormalities such as congenital diverticula or hiatus hernia may cause few, if any, symptoms even in later life.

# OESOPHAGEAL FOREIGN BODIES

The impaction of foreign bodies in the oesophagus is a common occurrence, the complications of which can be extremely serious and even life-threatening. The commonest objects to be swallowed are coins in children, and fish or meat bones in adults. Most objects that are swallowed pass harmlessly through the gut. However, sharp objects can stick in any part of the

## OVERVIEW
### Diseases of the Oesophagus

**Congenital**
- Stenosis
- Tracheo-oesophageal fistula
- Web

**Acquired**
**Foreign bodies**
- **Bolus**
- **Sharp**

**Trauma**
- Caustic (including gastro-oesophageal reflux)
- Rupture

**Infections**
- **Candida**

**Haematological disease**
- Patterson and Brown-Kelly syndrome – postcricoid web

**Neurological disease**
- Sensory failure
  lower cranial nerve palsies
- CNS and brainstem lesions
  motor neurone disease (MND), multiple sclerosis (MS), cerebrovascular accident (CVA), tumours, bulbar palsy, encephalitis, etc.
- PNS
  vagal neuroma, myasthenia gravis, achalasia

**Oesophageal tumours**
- Benign
- Malignant

**Connective tissue diseases**
- Scleroderma

**Degenerative conditions**
- Pharyngeal pouch
- **Hiatus hernia**

**Mechanical external compression**
- Hilar lymph nodes
- Cardiomegaly
- Thyroid enlargement

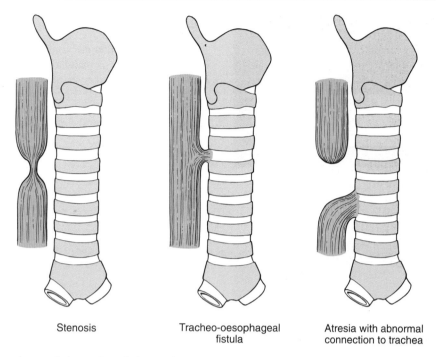

Stenosis | Tracheo-oesophageal fistula | Atresia with abnormal connection to trachea

FIGURE 6.1 Types of congenital oesophageal abnormalities.

gullet, and large food boluses can lodge in one of the natural narrowings of the oesophagus. If there is an oesophageal stricture, even small particles can impact and obstruct the oesophagus.

A good history is very helpful. In particular, one needs to establish whether or not there is, or could be, a bone or other sharp foreign body, since this will necessitate early intervention rather than a conservative course.

Particular features which are suggestive of a genuine foreign body are:

- The immediate onset of symptoms.
- Early presentation – within hours.
- Pain – retrosternal or back pain.
- A sense of a blockage in the throat.
- Drooling or regurgitation of food.
- Dyspnoea with or without hoarseness may occur if the object is lodged close to the larynx.
- Point tenderness in the neck.
- Discomfort on rocking the larynx from side to side.

## X-rays

Plain soft-tissue X-rays of the neck are often helpful (Figures 6.2 and 6.3); however, it must be remembered that some fish bones are radiolucent and will therefore not show up on plain X-ray. They may be localized when the patient is given a few shreds of cotton wool,

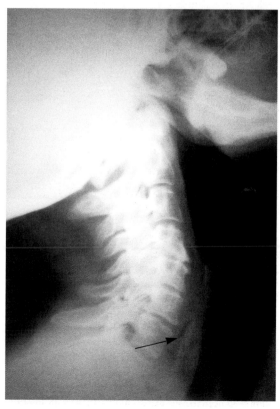

FIGURE 6.2 A lateral soft-tissue X-ray showing a bone lodged in the upper oesophagus.

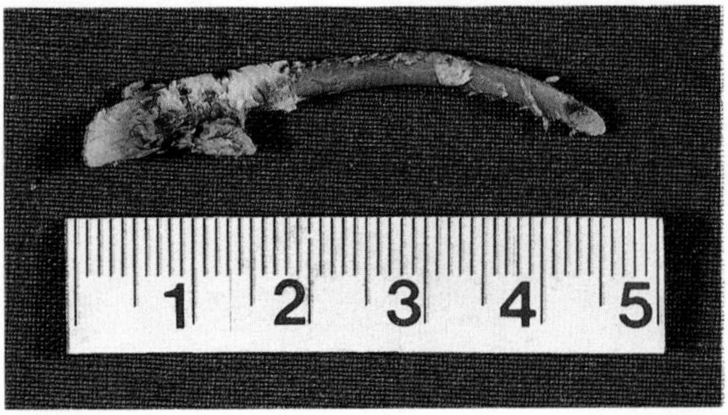

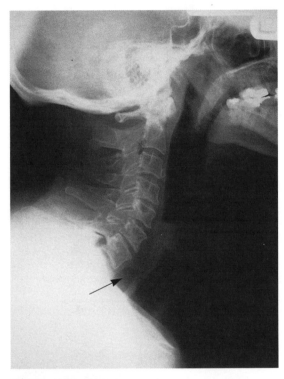

FIGURE 6.3 The bone removed.

FIGURE 6.4 Air in the upper oesophagus – a sign of an impacted foreign body.

soaked in barium. The cotton wool tends to catch on to the object.

Another suggestive feature is the presence of air in the upper oesophagus (Figure 6.4) or soft-tissue swelling of the posterior pharyngeal wall. Do not confuse the hyoid or thyroid cartilage with a foreign body, and remember that on X-ray, there are often flecks of calcification seen around the larynx. An oesophageal perforation will allow air to leak into the tissues of the neck. This, too, can be seen on an X-ray of the neck, usually in front of the spine.

## Treatment

Endoscopic removal under general anaesthesia is often required. Indeed, it is mandatory if there is any suggestion that the object is sharp, in which case there is a high risk of oesophageal perforation. In the case of a soft bolus obstruction, a *short* period of observation and treatment with intravenous antispasmodic agents *may* be indicated.

Potential complications are life-threatening and include para-oesophageal abscess, mediastinitis, empyema, airway obstruction, tracheo-oesophageal fistula and late stricture formation.

### KEY POINTS
#### Oesophageal Foreign Bodies

- A carefully taken history is paramount
- Lateral soft-tissue X-ray of the neck is often helpful
- Sharp foreign bodies should be removed at the earliest opportunity
- Soft foreign bodies may be treated conservatively for a short period
- Oesophageal foreign bodies can perforate the oesophagus

# GASTRO-OESOPHAGEAL REFLUX DISEASE (GORD) AND HIATUS HERNIA

## Symptoms

Mild, intermittent reflux of gastric contents into the oesophagus is common and often causes few, if any, symptoms. However, when severe, it is usually associated with a sliding hiatus hernia which results in an incompetent lower oesophageal sphincter. When affected patients lie down, stoop or strain, acidic gastric contents leak into the oesophagus. The oesophageal mucosa is damaged by gastric acid and inflammation and/or ulceration follows. Symptoms attributed to GORD include:

- Heartburn
- Retrosternal discomfort
- Nausea
- Waterbrash (bitter fluid regurgitating into the mouth)

When the condition is severe and prolonged, stricture formation and even malignant change have been described. Some controversy exists currently over some other conditions which have been attributed, at least by some experts, to GORD. These include globus pharyngeus, chronic laryngitis and even laryngeal neoplasia.

## Investigation

With the advent of effective medical therapy for GORD, many patients with classical histories are now given a therapeutic trial of either an $H_2$-receptor antagonist, e.g. ranitidine or cimetidine, or a proton pump inhibitor, e.g. omeprazole, prior to any investigation. In dubious or refractory cases, barium swallow, upper gastrointestinal endoscopy and 24-hour ambulatory oesophageal pH monitoring may be required in order to confirm the diagnosis.

## Treatment

Dietary, postural and medical therapy are the mainstays of treatment. Many patients are obese and losing weight is often effective in reducing symptoms. Patients should be advised to eat small frequent meals and avoid eating for a few hours before going to bed. Spicy foods, smoking and alcohol should also be discouraged. Avoiding bending and straining as well as propping up the head of the bed so as to reduce reflux at night, are all important strategies.

Medical treatment with antacids and alginates aims to neutralize the effects of excess acid production. $H_2$-blockers and omeprazole help to reduce the acid production. In very severe cases, surgical fundoplication may be required.

### KEY POINTS
#### GORD

- GORD is common
- Dietary and postural care are important and effective
- A therapeutic trial of medication is often effective
- Patients who fail a therapeutic trial should have malignancy excluded with endoscopy or barium swallow

# CAUSTIC INGESTION

Thankfully, accidental or intentional ingestion of corrosive substances is relatively rare. Bleach is the commonest offending agent. The victims are usually either children or have a psychiatric disturbance. They usually present in a state of shock with extensive chemical burns to the lips and mouth. The immediate threat is to the airway due to oedema and from mediastinitis as a result of oesophageal perforation.

Urgent advice from the National Poisons and Toxicology Unit should be sought. Intravenous fluids should be commenced and immediate oesophagoscopy arranged since this will allow assessment of the severity and extent of the injury as well as safe placement of a nasogastric tube. Broad-spectrum antibiotics and intravenous steroids are commenced. The injury is assessed at 10 days with direct endoscopy or barium swallow. A degree of stricture formation is likely and this will often require repeated dilations.

### CASE STUDY

Simon is a 29-year-old unemployed actor, who has noted a feeling of a lump in the throat for the last six months. He says, 'It feels like a pill has got stuck' and points to the area just below his larynx. His symptoms come and go and although food has never become stuck, he says that he sometimes finds it difficult to swallow his saliva. His grandfather died of carcinoma of the lung recently, and he admits that he is afraid that he has cancer. Examination is normal throughout.

1   What is the most likely diagnosis?
2   What other features should be sought on direct enquiry?
3   Should any investigations be organized? If so what?

**Comments**

1   This patient shows many of the features commonly found in globus pharyngeus.
2   A variety of associations are noted in this condition, e.g. gastro-oesophageal reflux, smoking, chronic sinusitis leading to postnasal drip, psychological stress and anxiety states. Each of these should be assessed.
3   After reassurance, many patients find their symptoms resolve. However, it is important to review each patient to ensure this is so. In those refractory cases, barium swallow and even direct endoscopy under general anaesthetic may be required in order to exclude an underlying neoplasia.

# NEUROLOGICAL CAUSES OF DYSPHAGIA

Swallowing is a dynamic and extremely complex reflex process which requires a sensory input, and a control centre within the CNS to receive this information and coordinate the motor side of the reflex arc. Any part of this reflex can be affected by disease and lead to swallowing problems.

The main *sensory* nerve supply of the pharynx is derived from the pharyngeal plexus, which is formed from branches of the IXth and Xth cranial nerves. The nucleus ambiguus in the brainstem serves as the *central coordinator*. The *motor* element to the pharyngeal muscles is from the cranial root of the XIth nerve. These fibres hitch-hike with the vagus on their way to the pharyngeal plexus.

The object of explaining this pathway is not so that the reader should try to remember the details, but so that he/she can appreciate that any lesion of the lower cranial nerves or brainstem can lead to problems on one or both sides of the reflex arc.

The lower cranial nerves exit through the base of the skull. Therefore tumours in this area will cause groups of palsies which can be recognized as clinical syndromes.

The commonest condition which affects the brainstem is a cerebrovascular accident. In this case, it is often fatal and problems with swallowing do not manifest themselves. Other conditions which affect the brainstem can lead to dysphagia, e.g. tumours, bulbar palsy, motor neurone disease, multiple sclerosis and infections such as encephalitis, polio and tabes dorsalis.

Difficulty in swallowing can also result from isolated cranial nerve lesions such as a vagal neuroma or systemic neurological disease such as myasthenia gravis.

## Assessment

Examination will reveal any cranial nerve palsy and a detailed swallowing history should help to identify if there are coughing or choking attacks with swallowing which may indicate aspiration into the respiratory tree. A chest X-ray may show collapse and consolidation of the lower lobes, particularly on the right side, if aspiration is a feature. A static picture of the swallowing process is gained by barium swallow. However, much more information is gained with dynamic video-swallow or fluoroscopy. This will not only show muscular incoordination of the oesophagus, but also any area of delay or pooling as well as overspill into the larynx. A speech and swallowing therapist should also be involved in the assessment of such patients, as should a dietician.

## Treatment

Many conditions are incurable or difficult to relieve and therefore treatment should be aimed at reducing symptoms by maximizing swallowing function and reducing aspiration. Initial treatment with swallowing therapy is vital prior to offering any of the following interventional treatment options:

- Swallowing therapy and dietary manipulation.
- Long-term nasogastric tube.
- Long-term feeding gastrostomy.
- Cricopharyngeal myotomy. This is performed to reduce the tone of the upper oesophageal sphincter.
- Vocal cord medialization in order to improve the cough reflex.
- Epiglottopexy aims to partially close off the larynx.
- Tracheostomy with insertion of a cuffed tube prevents laryngeal overspill reaching the larynx.
- Tracheal diversions or aryngectomy is a final resort.

# ACHALASIA

This is a rare condition in which there is a dilation of the lower oesophagus. The exact aetiology is uncertain but it is thought that a defect of the parasympathetic nerve plexus may be responsible. It is rather as if the lower oesophageal sphincter is hypertonic, but at endoscopy no increase in tension is found. The patient tends to be young and presents with progressive dysphagia, regurgitation and weight loss. Barium swallow is diagnostic (Figure 6.5) but endoscopy is also essential to exclude a coincident carcinoma. Treatment with inhaled amyl nitrate prior to meals may be effective. Otherwise, repeated dilation, cardioplasty or anastomotic procedures are required.

The condition should be differentiated from Chagas' disease which is caused by a treponemal infection leading to a similar dilation of the lower oesophagus.

# PHARYNGEAL POUCH

This is a type of hernia, or more accurately a pulsion-type diverticulum affecting the wall of the pharynx at its junction with the upper oesophagus. It occurs predominantly in men over the age of 50 years and is believed to result from an incoordination in the pharynx during swallowing, leading to an increased pharyngeal pressure above a 'closed' upper oesophageal

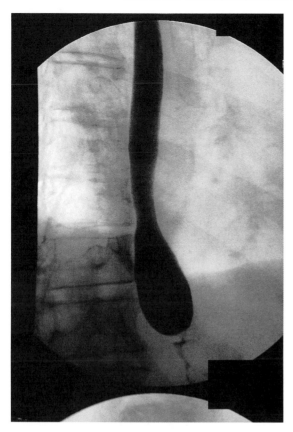

FIGURE 6.5 A barium swallow in achalasia.

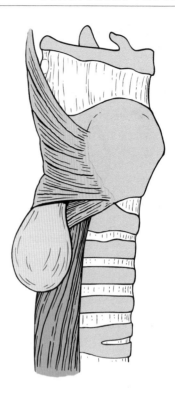

FIGURE 6.6 Pharyngeal mucosa herniating backwards through an area of weakness or Killian's dehiscence.

sphincter. As a result, the pharyngeal mucosa herinates backwards through a potential area of weakness, known as Killian's dehiscence (Figure 6.6). This is a potential space which arises between the two heads of the inferior constrictor muscle, namely its cricopharyngeal and thyropharyngeal components. The pouch initially develops posteriorly and then is deflected towards one side, nearly always the left.

## Presenting features

Features of a pharyngeal pouch include progressive dysphagia, regurgitation of undigested food, halitosis and gurgling noises emanating from the neck. Rarely, patients may present with a pneumonia as a result of otherwise silent laryngeal aspiration.

## Diagnosis

This is made on barium swallow (Figure 6.7) but rigid endoscopy should be performed to inspect the lining of the pouch and to exclude the rare finding of carcinoma arising within the pouch.

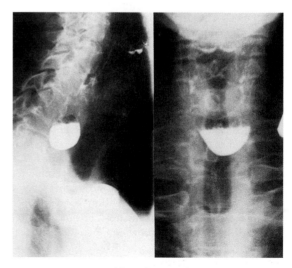

FIGURE 6.7 Anterior and lateral views of a pharyngeal pouch as seen on barium swallow. Published with the kind permission of Mr G. Bates FRCS.

## Treatment

This is only necessary if the patient is symptomatic. Various surgical options have been described and are

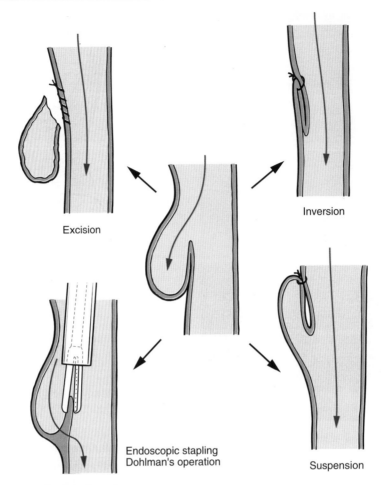

Excision

Inversion

Endoscopic stapling
Dohlman's operation

Suspension

FIGURE 6.8 Surgical options in pharyngeal pouch.

illustrated diagrammatically in Figure 6.8. Endoscopic division of the bar of tissue which divides the pouch from the oesophagus is achieved using diathermy or a laser. However, more recently, endoscopic stapling of pharyngeal pouches has rendered most other operations obsolete. In all cases, division of the upper oesophageal sphincter is mandatory in order to prevent recurrence. This is known as a cricopharyngeal myotomy.

## POSTCRICOID WEB

Patterson and Brown-Kelly were British and first described this condition in the UK. Plummer and Vinson were American and described the same disease in the USA. A web forms in the anterior upper oesophagus, behind the cricoid cartilage. This may cause dys-phagia and is visible on barium swallow. The other features of the syndrome include iron-deficiency or pernicious anaemia with koilonychia, atrophic glossitis and angular stomatitis. There is a small, but definite risk of malignant change in the postcricoid region, and as a result, all patients should have direct endoscopy, on a yearly basis if necessary. Treatment is that of the anaemia with endoscopic division of the web.

## OESOPHAGEAL TUMOURS

### Benign oesophageal tumours

Benign tumours of the oesophagus may arise from any of its tissue elements, e.g. leiomyoma, adenoma, lipoma, etc. All types are extremely rare and usually present with vague dysphagia.

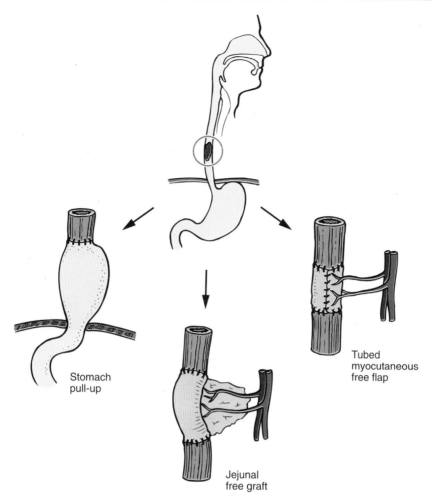

Stomach
pull-up

Jejunal
free graft

Tubed
myocutaneous
free flap

FIGURE 6.9 Surgical options in oesophageal cancer.

## CASE STUDY

Albert is 87 years old and, considering his age, was in good health until nine months ago. During this period, he has found he has some difficulty in swallowing his food. On occasions he has suffered with coughing fits during eating and drinking. He has lost 1 stone in weight over the last six months. Recently, rather to his disgust, he has regurgitated some undigested food which he remembers eating some days before.

1 What is the most likely diagnosis?
2 How will you confirm your diagnosis?
3 What are the treatment options?

### Comments
1 Obviously, a history of progressive dysphagia and weight loss in an elderly patient must raise the question of an oesophageal malignancy. However, in this case the diagnosis is that of a pharyngeal pouch.
2 Barium swallow will confirm the diagnosis.
3 Direct endoscopy in order to exclude an associated malignancy within the pouch is mandatory prior to any surgery. Thereafter, the pouch may be excised, inverted, suspended or even anastomosed to the oesophagus if massive. However, nowadays, the endoscopic stapling approach is safe, quick and effective and is the treatment of choice.

## Carcinoma of the oesophagus

Both squamous cell and adenocarcinomas occur in the oesophagus, most of the latter at the lower oesophageal junction. However, overall, about 50% of cancers arise in the middle third.

Over 80% of these tumours occur in males over the age of 60 years and affect the mid and lower two-thirds. In females, cancers occur most often in the upper third. Smoking, high alcohol intake, anaemia and achalasia are all predisposing factors.

Secondary metastatic deposits are very rare in the oesophagus but direct spread from bronchial, thyroid or stomach primaries may occur.

Progressive dysphagia, weight loss and discomfort in the throat are the common presenting features. Diagnosis is made on barium swallow and direct endoscopy.

Surgical excision may be curative if the tumour is small and has not escaped from the oesophagus. In this case, reconstruction of the defect with anastomosis is necessary. Various techniques are available. These include free jejunal grafting, stomach pull-up and myocutaneous flap reconstruction (Figure 6.9). With tumours of the upper oesophagus, laryngectomy is also required in order to gain adequate tumour clearance.

Palliative treatments include:

- Radiotherapy
- Laser debulking
- Intubation of a malignant stricture with a Celestin tube
- Bypass procedures
- Feeding gastrostomy

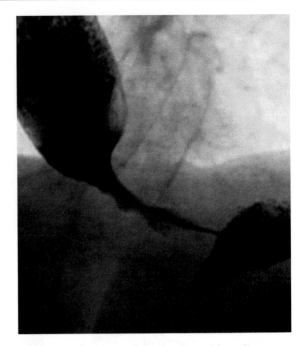

FIGURE 6.10 A barium swallow showing a tight malignant stricture at the gastro-oesophageal function.

## INVESTIGATION OF DYSPHAGIA

From the previous discussion, it can be seen that most causes of dysphagia can be diagnosed on barium swallow and/or endoscopy (Figure 6.10). A full blood count should be performed in order to exclude anaemia. In the case of suspected oesophageal cancers full pan-endoscopy must be performed in order to exclude another synchronous primary tumour.

Computed tomography (CT) and magnetic resonance imaging (MRI) scanning help to assess the extent of the tumour and aid the surgeon in deciding if the tumour is operable. Liver metastases should be excluded with an ultrasound scan prior to surgical intervention.

**KEY POINTS**
Dysphagia

- A detailed history often suggests the cause
- Look for cranial nerve palsies
- Barium swallow is diagnostic in most cases
- Remember that dysphagia and aspiration often occur together
- Aspiration is best assessed with videofluoroscopy
- Symptoms may be helped with swallowing therapy or surgical intervention
- Endoscopy is mandatory if cancers are suspected

# 7

# The thyroid gland

Clinical anatomy 72

Goitre 73

Neoplastic conditions of the thyroid 73

Investigation of thyroid disease 75

Treatment of thyroid conditions 76

Few other organs occupy so much attention, both in undergraduate and postgraduate exams. For this reason this chapter aims to give a fairly comprehensive surgical account of the gland and its disorders in order that the student be well equipped for combat!

## CLINICAL ANATOMY

The thyroid gland develops in embryo at the base of the tongue. It descends through the tissues of the anterior neck and finally comes to rest overlying the trachea and larynx (Figure 7.1). Faults in this process of descent can lead to congenital abnormalities such as a thyroglossal cyst (see page 84). The thyroid is enclosed by the pretracheal fascia and therefore it is bound to the trachea. As a result, the thyroid can be seen, or felt, to rise with the trachea and larynx as they ascend during swallowing.

The thyroid tissue is very vascular and consequently trauma to the thyroid (surgical or otherwise) can result in impressive bleeding into the neck. Also, bleeding into thyroid cysts is relatively common and this will lead to a rapid enlargement which is often painful due to stretching of the capsule of the gland.

The recurrent laryngeal nerves lie close to the back of each lobe of the gland as they pass upwards in the tracheo-oesophageal grooves to supply the vocal cords on each side. Thus, thyroid surgery or tumours of the gland may result in damage to these nerves which will result in a hoarse voice and a poor, 'breathy' cough. Malignant thyroid tumours can also invade the trachea, larynx or oesophagus and so lead to dysphagia, hoarseness or shortness of breath.

Great enlargement of the gland can occur with compression or displacement of the trachea. The gland may also enlarge downwards, into the chest – a so-called retrosternal extension. Here, the thyroid may have compressive effects on any of the mediastinal structures, most commonly the great veins, which subsequently leads to venous engorgement of the neck. Usually during examination of a normal neck, the thyroid gland will be neither seen nor felt.

Thyroid surgery is generally performed either by general or ENT surgeons. However, it must be recognized that whichever specialty is performing this surgery, they must also work closely with an endocrinologist, preferably in a dedicated joint clinic.

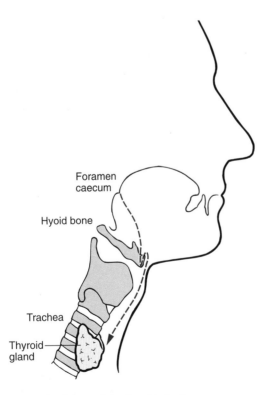

FIGURE 7.1 The descent of the thyroid gland.

**OVERVIEW**
Diseases of the Thyroid Gland

**Infective**
- De Quervain's thyroiditis

**Autoimmune**
- **Hashimoto's Thyroiditis**
- **Graves' disease**

**Neoplastic**
*Benign*
- **Adenoma**
*Malignant*
- **Papillary adenocarcinoma**
- **Follicular adenocarcinoma**
- Medullary carcinoma
- Anaplastic carcinoma
- Lymphoma
- Hürtle cell tumour

**Endocrine**
- **Physiological goitre** of adolescence or pregnancy
- Simple (iodine-deficiency) goitre

**Degenerative**
- Simple cysts
- **Multinodular goitre**

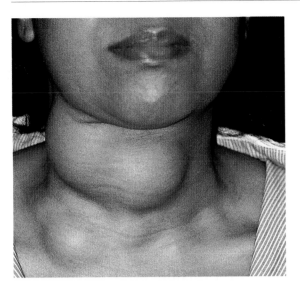

FIGURE 7.2 A goitre.

# GOITRE (Figure 7.2)

Goitre means swelling or enlargement of the thyroid gland. It is a descriptive term only and is not a diagnosis. Both physiological and pathological conditions may cause a goitre.

## Diffuse enlargement of the thyroid

This may occur either as a result of dietary iodine deficiency (simple goitre) or may occur in pregnancy where it is described as a physiological goitre. In Graves' disease autoantibodies are formed which mimic the effect of thyroid-stimulating hormone (TSH) to stimulate the gland excessively. As a result, the gland undergoes diffuse enlargement.

## Nodular enlargement of the thyroid

In some cases, the thyroid gland may undergo nodular, rather than a smooth, enlargement. A *single or solitary* nodule within the thyroid must raise the question of a malignancy and should be managed as outlined below. Multiple nodules may arise within the gland in response to alternating episodes of thyroid hormone deficiency and subsequent TSH hypersecretion. This is followed by hyperplasia of the gland. Such prolonged periods of hyperplasia and involution over prolonged periods cause nodularity. The resulting *multinodular goitre* results from periods of dietary iodine deficiency, or may arise sporadically. In such a

case, thyroidectomy is only necessary in order to rectify cosmetic or compressive symptoms.

# NEOPLASTIC CONDITIONS OF THE THYROID

Histological examination of thyroid tissue shows the gland to be composed largely of follicles and supporting

## CASE STUDY

Jenny is 58 years old and complains that her 'neck is getting fat'. She offers no other symptoms but does admit to a slight feeling of a lump in her throat, particularly on swallowing. On examination she has a bilobed midline mass which moves on swallowing. This is smooth and non-tender. The rest of her examination is normal. An ultrasound scan is ordered which confirms the clinical suspicion of an enlarged thyroid gland. Furthermore, the gland has a multinodular structure.

1   What is the diagnosis?
2   At what point should surgery be considered?
3   What are the major risks of thyroid surgery?

**Comments**
1   Multinodular goitre.
2   If the patient develops compressive or cosmetic symptoms, one may consider thyroid surgery. Also, if there is any suspicion of an associated malignancy, either at presentation or in the follow-up period.
3   The recurrent laryngeal nerves are closely related to the posterior part of the thyroid gland and damage to one of these structures may lead to a hoarse voice. If bilateral palsy results, the patient may develop stridor. The other main risk of thyroid surgery is of a reactionary haemorrhage. Here, a neck haematoma may develop with frightening speed and the patient may once again develop airway problems as a result of tracheal compression. Immediate opening of the wound, aspiration of the haematoma and control of the bleeding point is required, on the ward if necessary. The parathyroid glands may also be damaged at surgery and postoperative hypocalcaemia may develop. In the longer term, hypothyroidism may develop following thyroid surgery.

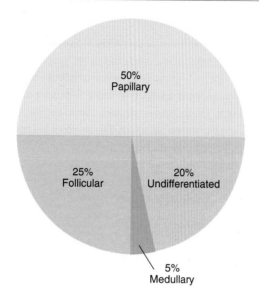

FIGURE 7.3 Distribution of thyroid tumours.

cells. Tumours of the thyroid may arise from either of these cellular elements, but the vast majority of such neoplasms arise from the follicular cells and three different types of tumour result: papillary, follicular and anaplastic carcinomas. The supporting, or parafollicular cells, give rise to medullary carcinomas. Each variety of tumour has its own particular characteristics and behaviour (Figure 7.3).

## Papillary adenocarcinoma

This tumour can arise at any age but is most common between the ages of 40 and 50 years. These tumours tend to be multifocal, with multiple primary tumours within the gland; 60% of patients have clinically involved neck nodes at presentation. When the disease is confined to the thyroid, ten-year survival rates are excellent (90%); however, if tumour has spread to the lymph nodes, the prognosis is less good (60%).

Since the tumour is frequently multifocal, near total thyroidectomy is the treatment of choice, with a neck dissection if there is lymphatic spread. Postoperatively, radioactive iodine is given to ablate any viable thyroid which is left behind; obviously thyroid hormone replacements will be required long term.

## Follicular adenocarcinoma

Here, the patients tend to be older, most being between the ages of 50 and 60 years. The tumours tend to have a well-defined capsule. These tumours, rather than spreading via the lymph system, tend to spread haematogenously, and 30% of patients will have bony metastases which readily take up iodine. The treatment is similar to that for the papillary variety.

## Anaplastic carcinoma

This is a deadly tumour from which 92% of patients will die within one year despite treatment. It tends to affect elderly women, particularly where there has been long-standing thyroid enlargement. Patients present with a rapidly enlarging mass, pain, referred otalgia and symptoms due to invasion of the larynx, trachea or oesophagus. Radical radiotherapy offers the only hope of cure; however, early recurrence is the rule.

## Medullary carcinoma

This occurs in the multiple endocrine neoplasia (MEN) syndrome. The tumour arises from the parafollicular C cells, which secrete calcitonin. As a result, the plasma levels of this hormone are raised. However, the serum level of calcium remains normal. Regional lymph nodes are affected in approximately 30% of cases. Treatment comprises near total thyroidectomy and radiotherapy.

## Benign adenoma

A benign tumour of the thyroid may, or may not, secrete thyroxine. An actively secreting tumour will take up radioactive iodine or technetium and is known as a 'hot' nodule. Symptoms of thyrotoxicosis may develop. If a hot nodule fails to respond to thyroxine suppressive treatment, it should either be excised or ablated with radioiodine. Hot nodules are rarely malignant.

Non-functioning adenomas also occur; these do not take up iodine and are known as 'cold' nodules; 10–20% of cold nodules will, in fact, represent a malignant rather than a benign tumour, and these therefore require further investigation as outlined below.

> **KEY POINTS**
> ### Thyroid and Related Swellings
>
> - Thyroid lumps move on swallowing
> - Thyroglossal tract remnants move on protruding the tongue (see page 84)
> - When presented with a thyroid swelling, try to determine if it is a diffuse enlargement of the gland, a multinodular goitre or a single lump within the gland

# INVESTIGATION OF THYROID DISEASE

Obviously, prior to any investigation, a complete history and examination must be obtained. In particular, any signs or symptoms of thyroid over- or underactivity must be elicited (Tables 7.1 and 7.2). The commonly performed thyroid investigations and their indications are presented here. However, the reader should be aware that it is most unlikely that it will be necessary to perform all of these tests in every patient. In Figure 7.4, we suggest a scheme for the investigation and management of a lump in the thyroid gland.

TABLE 7.1  Signs and symptoms of thyroid disease

| Hyperthyroidism | Hypothyroidism |
| --- | --- |
| Irritability | Mental slowness |
| Heat intolerance | Cold intolerance |
| Insomnia | Hypersomnolence |
| Sweaty skin | Dry skin |
| Amenorrhoea | Menorrhagia |
| Weight loss | Weight gain |
| Diarrhoea | Constipation |
| Palpitations | Bradycardia |
| Hyper-reflexia | Slow relaxing reflexes |
| Tremor | Loss of outer third of eyebrow |
| Atrial fibrillation | Hoarse voice |

TABLE 7.2  Thyroid eye signs (Graves' disease)

| Lid lag | Lid retraction |
| --- | --- |
| Exophthalmos | Proptosis |
| Ophthalmoplegia | Chemosis |

## Blood tests

### Thyroid function tests

Thyroxine ($T_4$) and its more active product, tri-iodothyronine ($T_3$), are carried in the bloodstream where they are mainly bound to plasma proteins. However, a proportion remains unbound, and it is this 'free' component which is physiologically active. The clinical relevance of this fact is that false results may be obtained in situations where this free-to-bound balance is disturbed, for example when plasma proteins are low as in the nephrotic syndrome or high as in pregnancy. Using modern radioimmunoassay techniques, the levels of free $T_3$ and $T_4$ can be determined directly. The levels of thyroid-stimulating hormone (TSH), which stimulates the release of thyroid hormones from the gland, are controlled by a negative feedback mechanism acting on the

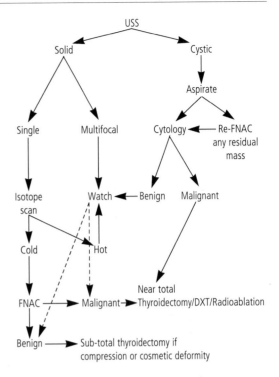

FIGURE 7.4 Flowchart for the investigation and management of a thyroid lump.

hypothalamus. Thus TSH levels are usually raised in hypothyroidism and depressed in hyperthyroidism.

## Thyroglobulin

This is a carrier protein for thyroxine. Its level can be measured, and is used as a tumour marker for differentiated thyroid tumours.

## Carcinoembryonic antigen (CEA)

This is used as a marker of medullary carcinomas of the thyroid.

## Calcitonin

This is produced by the medullary C cells and therefore is also raised in medullary carcinomas of the thyroid gland.

## Thyroid autoantibodies

These are found in autoimmune conditions such as Hashimoto's and Graves' disease.

## Thyroid radioisotope scanning

An oral dose of radioactive iodine ($^{123}$I) or technetium ($^{99}$Tc) is given and its subsequent uptake into metabolically active thyroid tissue measured. This investigation is used in the assessment of a solitary thyroid nodule. If it takes up the iodine, the nodule is described as 'hot'; if not, then it is called 'cold'; 80% of such nodules are cold and 10–20% of these will be malignant. Nearly all hot nodules are benign.

Isotope scanning is also very useful in the assessment of malignant thyroid metastases or ectopic thyroid tissue.

## Ultrasound (USS)

Ultrasound is excellent at distinguishing solid from cystic structures and frequently will show that what feels clinically like a solitary lump, is in fact part of a multinodular goitre. It has no use in the diagnosis of malignancy, but ultrasound-guided fine-needle aspiration cytology (FNAC) can be useful in this regard.

## Computed tomography (CT) and magnetic resonance imaging (MRI) scanning

These are useful in the assessment of a retrosternal goitre since they show the extent of the gland's descent into the chest and its relationship to the important mediastinal structures. Compression or displacement of the trachea is also well demonstrated. In locally invasive, malignant thyroid tumours, the site and degree of invasion may be determined using these scanning techniques.

## Fine-needle aspiration cytology (FNAC)

This can be an extremely useful investigation, since a result which confirms a malignancy will aid in planning further treatment. Also, when a benign result is achieved, surgery may be avoided altogether. In experienced hands, the technique can reliably diagnose most causes of a thyroid lump. However, it does have its limitations. For example, it is impossible to differentiate a follicular adenoma from a follicular carcinoma, since this relies upon the demonstration of capsular invasion which is not possible with this technique. Cystic lesions should have a repeat FNAC once aspirated, in order to biopsy the residual lump. A cystic lesion should be excised if the cytology is suspicious or if the cyst re-accumulates.

# TREATMENT OF THYROID CONDITIONS

## Hormonal manipulation

In cases of hypothyroidism, thyroxine replacements are required on a daily basis; after thyroidectomy, such treatment is mandatory life-long. Thyroxine is also administered as a part of treatment for some thyroid tumours, in an attempt to suppress the growth of these hormone-dependent neoplasms.

Propylthiouracil and carbimazole inhibit the formation of the thyroid hormones and are used in cases of hyperthyroidism.

## Radioactive ablation

Some types of thyroid tumours trap iodine and this ability can be determined via an isotope scan. After thyroidectomy for a malignant tumour, any residual or metastatic thyroid tissue will readily trap iodine in response to the raised TSH levels which ensue. This mechanism is put to good use by administering radioactive iodine in the hope that the tumour tissue will concentrate a lethal dose of radiation.

In some cases of hyperthyroidism which are unresponsive to medical treatment, the thyroid tissue is ablated in the same way.

## Thyroid surgery

Hemi-, near total and total thyroidectomy are the operations most often performed. Which of these is required will depend on the underlying disease and its extent.

Hemithyroidectomy involves removal of one lobe of the thyroid gland. This is usually performed for benign conditions and in low-grade malignancies. Total thyroidectomy is performed in cases of malignancy; however, the risk of damage to the recurrent laryngeal nerves and the potential complications of hypoparathyroidism which will inevitably occur, lead many surgeons to favour a near total excision. This leaves a small remnant of thyroid bilaterally which will preserve the parathyroid glands and also reduce the risk to the recurrent laryngeal nerve.

Prior to surgery the patient must be warned of the potential for permanent recurrent laryngeal nerve palsy and it is routine practice for the patient to have a 'cord check' before their surgery in order to document the mobility of the vocal folds for medico-legal reasons. If the cords are paralysed as a result of recurrent laryngeal nerve damage during thyroid surgery, there is a risk of life-threatening airway obstruction. Therefore, in all cases, facilities for intubation and tracheostomy must be available in the recovery area and on the ward.

Where the parathyroid glands have been removed or disturbed, there is a risk of hypocalcaemia in the early post-operative period. Therefore, the corrected serum calcium levels must be checked regularly and replacements given where necessary.

> **KEY POINTS**
> ## Treatment of Thyroid Conditions
>
> - Malignant thyroid lumps should be surgically removed
> - Benign thyroid lumps should be surgically removed if there are compressive or cosmetic defects
> - The recurrent laryngeal nerve is at risk during thyroid surgery
> - Pre-operative vocal cord check is required for medico-legal reasons before thyroid surgery
> - Radioactive ablation is used to destroy the last vestiges of thyroid tissue after removal of a thyroid malignancy, and also to ablate an overactive thyroid gland which is unresponsive to medical treatment

# 8

# The neck

Clinical anatomy of the neck  80

Investigation of neck lumps  82

Congenital neck remnants  84

Neck infections  86

Lymph node enlargement  86

Neck hernias  87

# CLINICAL ANATOMY OF THE NECK

## Surface anatomy

The sternomastoid muscle divides the neck into two anatomical triangles. These are often referred to in clinical practice (*and also in exams*) when describing lumps in the neck and therefore an understanding of these is essential. It should be recognized that these triangles are artificial and have not been chosen for clinical or embryological reasons and as a result pathology does not often respect or follow their boundaries (Figure 8.1).

Using Figure 8.2 try to identify the position of all the following important structures on yourself:

(a) Mastoid process
(b) Heads of the clavicles
(c) Sternomastoid muscle
(d) Trachea
(e) Cricoid cartilage
(f) Cricothyroid membrane
(g) Thyroid prominence
(h) Hyoid bone
(i) Carotid artery bifurcation
(j) Thyroid gland
(k) Parotid gland
(l) Submandibular gland
(m) Jugulodigastric lymph node

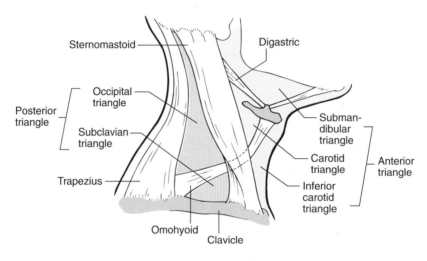

FIGURE 8.1 Triangles of the neck.

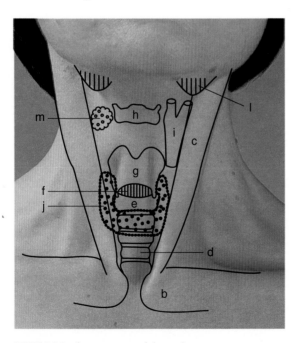
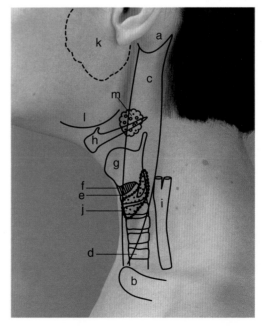

FIGURE 8.2 Surface anatomy of the neck.

Don't be alarmed if you feel one or two small, soft lymph glands. It is quite a common finding in normal people, especially in children. There are 200–300 lymph nodes in a normal person's head and neck. The largest and most frequently enlarged is the jugulodigastric node.

## Deep neck anatomy

The neck is divided into anatomical compartments by strong fascia which is arranged in layers and tends to align neck structures in bundles. These are real and important anatomical divisions and have great relevance clinically.

Broadly speaking, where the fascial planes of the neck cross a bony structure, such as the hyoid, they are fused to it. The outermost layer which surrounds the neck is the investing fascia. This is often described as similar to a polo-neck jumper. It is attached above to the mandible and skull base and below to the clavicles and cervical spine. More fascial planes divide the neck into compartments.

There are two main compartments of the neck which are separated by the prevertebral fascia (Figure 8.3):

- The *posterior, skeletal compartment* which contains the cervical spine and its musculature. This need concern us no further.
- The *anterior, visceral compartment* which contains all the other structures and organs. It contains bundles of structures each of which is enclosed by a fascial envelope (Figure. 8.4). The most important of these are:

The *pretracheal fascia* is clinically relevant since it encloses the thyroid gland and binds it to the trachea. Thus, when the larynx and trachea move with swallowing, the thyroid gland also ascends and descends.

The *carotid sheath*. This is a fascial bundle which encloses the carotid, internal jugular vein and vagus nerve.

### OVERVIEW
### Neck Diseases

**Congenital**
- **Branchial cyst**
- **Thyroglossal cysts**
- Cystic hygroma
- Dermoid cyst

**Acquired**
**Skin and subcutaneous tissue**
- **Sebaceous cysts**
- **Lipomas**
- **Furuncle**

**Lymph nodes**
- Benign
  **general: reactive lymphadenitis**
  specific infections: **glandular fever**: HIV, TB, toxoplasmosis, etc.
- Malignant
  **primary**
  **metastatic**

**Blood vessels**
- Carotid body tumours
- Carotid aneurysm

**Nerves**
- Vagal neuroma

**Salivary glands**
- **Sialadenitis/sialolithiasis**
- Tumours: benign and malignant

**Larynx**
- External laryngocoele

**Pharynx**
- Pharyngeal pouch

**Thyroid**
- **Simple/physiological goitre**
- **Solitary nodule**
- **Multinodular goitre**
- **Thyroid tumours: benign and malignant**
- Thyroiditis

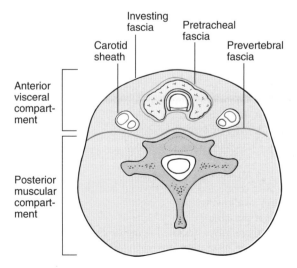

FIGURE 8.3 Fascial layers of the neck.

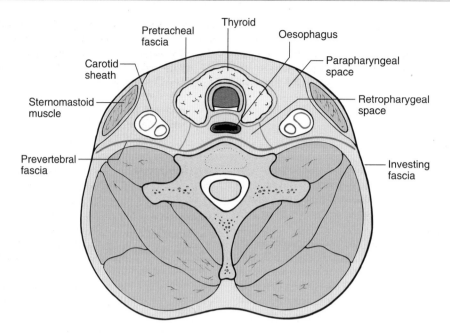

FIGURE 8.4 Fascial layers and spaces of the neck.

Between all of the fascial bundles are potential spaces, known collectively as the deep neck spaces. Herein lies further clinical relevance since disease, particularly infections of the neck, can spread along these spaces to form deep-seated abscesses. The most important of the named deep neck spaces are the parapharyngeal, retropharyngeal and submandibular (Figure 8.5).

# INVESTIGATION OF NECK LUMPS

## Making the clinical diagnosis

A good history and careful examination will often point to a clinical diagnosis, which will in turn help to guide towards ordering the appropriate investigations necessary to confirm the diagnosis. The duration of the history and the presence of any intercurrent illness are important factors to ascertain. A history of pain and/or swelling in a neck lump usually indicates an inflammatory process, and if these symptoms are clearly related to eating, then sialadenitis/sialolithiasis must be suspected.

When examining the patient, try to answer the following questions in order to determine the lump's characteristics:

- What is its site?
- What is its size?
- What is its shape?

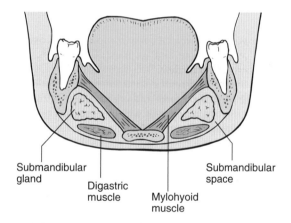

FIGURE 8.5 The submandibular space.

- Is it smooth or lobulated?
- Is it in the midline?
- Is it solid or cystic?
- Is there more than one lump?
- Is it tender?
- Is it attached to any viscus?
- Is it connected to the thyroid and therefore moves on swallowing?
- Is it pulsatile ?
- Is there any associated acute or chronic inflammation or ulceration anywhere within the head and neck? (Remember this includes the scalp, oral and nasal cavities.)

# Confirmatory investigations

Having arrived at a clinical diagnosis, or at least a list of differential diagnoses, one usually needs to perform confirmatory investigations. Obviously these will vary depending on the most likely cause of the lump.

## Blood tests

Full blood count (FBC) is frequently performed. Occasionally it is diagnostic. However, more often it contributes to, or detracts from, a diagnosis. For example, a raised white cell count suggests an infective process. Similarly, the erythrocyte sedimentation rate (ESR) is rarely diagnostic in itself but often helpful nevertheless.

## Monospot or Paul Bunnell test

This will confirm that generalized lymphadenopathy is due to glandular fever (infectious mononucleosis). Remember, also, to examine the axillae and groins as well as checking for liver and spleen enlargement.

## HIV

HIV testing and other serum tests for specific infections such as toxoplasmosis are sometimes necessary in cases of chronic generalized lymphadenopathy.

## Radiology

A chest X-ray (CXR) is often indicated both where malignancy and chronic benign lymphadenopathy are suspected. An ultrasound scan (USS) is helpful in some circumstances. It is particularly good at distinguishing between cystic and solid lumps. USS is the investigation of choice in the thyroid gland and is also very useful in diagnosing vascular lesions. Computed tomography (CT) and magnetic resonance imaging (MRI) scanning are being used more and more frequently, especially in tumours of the head and neck. It should be realized that they are rarely diagnostic but may be helpful by demonstrating the anatomy and extent of the lesion.

## Cytology

Fine-needle aspiration cytology (FNAC) is extremely useful in diagnosing the cause of many lumps in the neck. It is important to recognize that interpreting samples from this technique is difficult and demands an experienced cytologist. Also, some tissues are diffi-cult to decipher accurately. For example, thyroid lumps and lymphomas. However, it is simple and cheap to perform. Also, it can be carried out by a doctor in the clinic with ease. For these reasons we describe the technique in detail.

### Fine-needle aspiration cytology

The procedure is explained to the patient who is asked to lie down on a couch. The skin is cleaned and the lump fixed firmly with the fingers. A green (22G) needle is attached to a 10-ml syringe. The needle is passed through the skin to the approximate centre of the lump. At this point, suction is applied to the syringe by withdrawing the plunger (a syringe holder greatly facilitates this otherwise awkward one-handed procedure).

Now, with suction applied, the needle is passed repeatedly backwards and forwards through the lump. As a result, cells are drawn up into the barrel of the needle. If at any time blood should 'flash back' into the syringe, the sample should be regarded as contaminated and the procedure repeated. Four to six passes through the lump should give an adequate sample in most cases. The suction must be released prior to withdrawing the syringe. This is to avoid contamination of the sample with skin cells.

The needle is removed and the syringe filled with air. Then the needle is replaced and its contents are expelled onto a clean glass slide. This manoeuvre should be repeated several times until no more material can be expelled. The sample material is then spread as thinly as possible over the slide which is then labelled, fixed and left to dry.

## Endoscopy

Carcinomas which arise in the head and neck often metastasise to the regional lymph nodes in the neck. Therefore, when a patient presents with such a node, an examination of the possible primary sites is essential since this tumour must be identified and treated if the patient is to survive. With the advent of fibreoptic endoscopes, many of the potential sites of tumour genesis can be visualized in the ENT outpatients. However, it is not possible to take biopsies easily and some areas remain hidden. For these reasons pan-endoscopy is performed under general anaesthesia. If no obvious tumour is seen, 'blind' biopsies are taken from the likely sites:

- Nasopharynx
- Tongue base
- Tonsil
- Vallecula
- Pyriform fossae
- Postcricoid region

## Biopsy

In some cases, the origin or the exact nature of a neck lump cannot be identified using the above investigations. In this case, open biopsy of the neck lump is required. As a general rule, such a biopsy should be *excisional*, rather than *incisional*, since here there is a danger of a tumour spreading to a previously uninvolved area. This can result in compromising further treatment. In order accurately to diagnose the various types of lymphoma, the ENT surgeon will often need to perform such an excisional biopsy since it is the detailed micro-architecture of the node which proves diagnostic in subtyping lymphomas.

# CONGENITAL NECK REMNANTS

## Thyroglossal cyst and fistula

These lesions, although congenital, do not often present at birth, but more commonly in childhood or early adulthood. They result from defects in the development of the thyroid gland. The thyroid develops at the tongue base and in embryo descends downwards, around or through the hyoid bone, and through the tissues of the neck, to eventually overlie the trachea and thyroid cartilage (see Figure 7.1, page 72). As a result of this descent, a tract is left which runs from the foramen caecum of the tongue to the thyroid gland. The tract usually resorbs, however; if it remains, cyst or fistula formation of the tract can result (Figure 8.6).

The lesions are virtually always present in the midline and will move upwards when the patient sticks out their tongue, due to the attachment of the tract to the hyoid and tongue base. The patient may notice a swelling, or, in the case of a fistula may complain of a discharging area at the front of the neck. In fact, spontaneous fistula formation is rare and usually results from misguided attempts to drain an abscess or other surgical intervention.

Treatment consists of surgical excision of the whole tract, including the body of the hyoid bone. Attempts at local excision of these defects are misguided since the problem will often recur unless the whole tract is removed, from neck skin to tongue base if necessary.

## Branchial cyst and fistulae

### Branchial cyst

Once again, these tend to present before the age of 30 years, and occur in a characteristic position. They

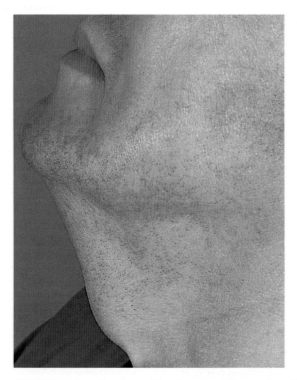
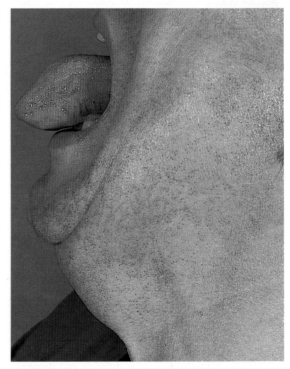

FIGURE 8.6 A thyroglossal cyst. Note how the midline neck swelling ascends when the tongue is protruded.

present with a lump in the neck situated in the region of the middle third of the sternomastoid muscle (Figure 8.7). If the cyst becomes infected, it may be painful.

It was largely accepted that these lesions arose as a result of an abnormality of fusion of the embryological branchial clefts. However, more recently, it has been suggested that they may result from epithelial inclusions within a lymph node which later undergoes a process of cystic degeneration.

Enlarged lymph nodes of the deep cervical chain, and other laterally based neck swellings may lead to diagnostic difficulty, but in the case of a branchial cyst FNAC will result in a pus-like aspirate which is rich in cholesterol crystals (Figure 8.8). Treatment is by surgical excision.

## Branchial fistulae

These occur as a result of defects in fusion of the branchial clefts. Here, a fistula tract runs from the

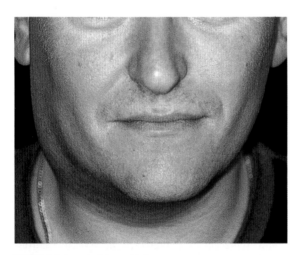

FIGURE 8.7 A typical branchial cyst.

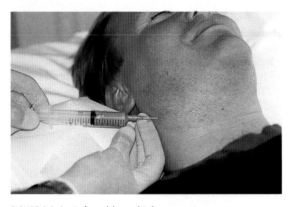

FIGURE 8.8 An infected branchial cyst aspirate.

## CASE STUDY

Adam, a 27-year-old surveyor, presents complaining of a lump on the right side of his neck. It came up rapidly three weeks ago, and since then has increased and decreased in size slightly, but has not gone away. He feels well in himself and examination reveals a 4 cm × 3 cm swelling, just deep to the upper third of the sternomastoid muscle on the right side. It is a little tender and has a smooth surface. It is rubbery in consistency and appears fluctuant. It does not transilluminate.

1  What is the diagnosis?
2  What investigation would you perform?
3  How is this condition treated?

### Comments

1  In a young patient, a rapidly enlarging neck swelling, especially with the features of a cyst, is very likely to represent a branchial cyst.
2  Fine-needle aspiration will reveal fluid which may be purulent if the cyst has become infected. Cytological examination of the aspirate is usually diagnostic.
3  Surgical excision.

skin, usually at a site close to the anterior border of the sternomastoid muscle, to the tonsillar fossa. It passes between the great arteries and veins of the neck, in close proximity to the lower cranial nerves. Surgical excision is demanding as it involves dissection between these structures.

## Dermoids

These, again, result from defects of fusion in embryo, but here elements of the skin become trapped subcutaneously and develop into cysts which are lined with squamous epithelium and skin appendages such as hair follicles and sweat glands. They present as painless midline swellings anywhere between the suprasternal notch and the chin, but unlike thyroid remnants, they do not move on swallowing or protrusion of the tongue. Complete surgical excision is the only treatment.

## Cystic hygroma

A cystic hygroma is a rare type of lymphangioma, i.e. benign tumours of lymph vessels. Lymphangiomas in general are classified according to the size of the vessels within the tumour. Capillary and cavernous lymphangiomas consist of small and medium-sized vessels, respectively.

Cystic hygroma is the name given to these tumours when the vessels are very large and dilated. They occur in the neck and expand between the tissue planes. They are usually noticed at, or soon after, birth and may be very large in which case vital structures within the neck, e.g. the trachea may be compressed. Staged, multiple excisions are sometimes needed over many years.

# NECK INFECTIONS

## Parapharyngeal abscess

This is a rare infection of the parapharyngeal space (see page 82) and usually results from lower jaw dental infection or tonsillitis. The patient is pyrexial, toxic and has a neck swelling which is usually slightly behind the sternomastoid. They have trismus and the tonsil is pushed medially. If the patient does not respond to intravenous antibiotics after 48 hours, surgical drainage of the space is essential.

## Ludwig's angina

Here, the submandibular space is affected. It usually results from dental infection with *Streptococcus viridans* being the pathogen most frequently isolated. The patient is pyrexial, drooling, has trismus and may suffer from airway obstruction due to backward displacement of the tongue. There is a firm swelling of the tissues of the floor of mouth. First-line treatment is with intravenous antibiotics since incision seldom finds pus. If the airway is threatened, a tracheostomy may be required.

# LYMPH NODE ENLARGEMENT

The function of the lymph nodes within the head and neck, as anywhere in the body, is to provide a local defence mechanism against infection or tumour. When active, the nodes enlarge and become palpable.

## Infective lymphadenopathy

When the nodes enlarge as a result of infection they are usually tender. Often the site of the infection is obvious, e.g. tonsillitis. However, occasionally one or

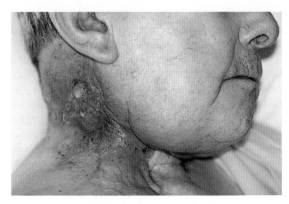

FIGURE 8.9 A squamous cell carcinoma fungating through the skin despite previous radiotherapy and neck dissection.

more nodes may enlarge without any obvious primary infected site. In this case, one must consider specific infections such as infectious mononucleosis, tuberculosis, HIV, toxoplasmosis, actinomycosis, brucellosis and cat-scratch fever.

## Neoplastic lymphadenopathy

Malignancy must be excluded when an enlarging, or persistently, palpable lymph node is present in an adult. In early adulthood, the most likely neoplasm is a lymphoma which may require excisional biopsy. In the older patient, there is a higher chance that a malignant node contains squamous cell carcinoma (Figure 8.9). This will have originated from a primary tumour somewhere within the head and neck, and in some cases may be microscopic and asymptomatic. These metastatic squamous deposits are usually easy to diagnose on FNAC.

As already stated, all patients in whom a neck lump could represent a malignancy deserve a rigorous search for the primary site and this *must* begin with referral to an ENT clinic where facilities for a full examination of the head and neck are available. From this initial examination, the primary site may well be evident. However, not infrequently, a small primary may remain elusive. In this case a full examination of all these areas must be performed under anaesthetic with 'blind' biopsies of those areas under suspicion.

The TNM classification is used to stage metastatic nodes in the neck. Based on this staging and the site and size of the primary tumour, a treatment plan can be decided upon.

| | |
|---|---|
| N1 | Single node, ipsilateral, < 3 cm |
| N2 | Single node, ipsilateral > 3 cm and < 6 cm or multiple ipsilateral nodes < 6 cm or contralateral nodes < 6 cm |
| N3 | Any node > 6 cm |

The treatment options in squamous cell carcinomas of the head and neck usually consist of either radiotherapy or surgery, and not infrequently a combination of the two. The basic surgical approach is that of radical excision of the primary tumour with *en bloc* resection of the affected nodes via a neck dissection. The basic aim of a *radical neck dissection* is to remove all the lymph-bearing structures which lie between the skull base and clavicle. This necessitates sacrificing the sternomastoid, internal jugular vein and accessory nerve. Modifications of this operation with preservation of some or all of the above structures, and selective dissections of groups of affected lymph nodes are also employed in some cases.

# NECK HERNIAS

## Laryngocoele

The characteristic bulging neck of the bullfrog is well known to most of us. It is due to inflation of an air sac which is connected to its airway. In fact, many lower animals have similar air sacs. It is thought that a small blind ending space, called the saccule, found in the human larynx, may represent this vestigial structure. Sometimes the saccule can enlarge to produce a laryngocoele. This is a blind ending out pouching of the laryngeal mucosa. Laryngocoeles, as they expand, may remain enclosed within the framework of the larynx, in which case they are known as an *internal laryngocoele*. Alternatively, they can escape from the larynx, via a potential weak spot in the thyrohyoid membrane where the superior laryngeal neurovascular bundle pierces this layer. In this case, the abnormality is described as an *external laryngocoele*. An external laryngocoele may present as a lump in the neck, usually in association with hoarseness.

It has been postulated that this condition is more common in glassblowers and trumpet players. However, there is little evidence to support this. It is more important to recognize that a small carcinoma at the site of the neck of the saccule can lead to a valve-like effect with subsequent laryngocoele development. Once this has been excluded, treatment is by surgical excision of the sac and repair of the defect, as in any hernia repair.

## Pharyngeal pouch

This is another type of herniation or pulsion diverticula. Here, the mucosa of the upper oesophagus herinates through a potential weak spot in constrictor muscles of the pharynx, known as Killian's dehiscence. This more frequently causes swallowing problems, but can also present as a lump in the neck. We have discussed this condition more fully in Chapter 6.

Conditions of the salivary glands and thyroid may present with a lump in the neck. However, these conditions are also dealt with in more detail in other chapters.

---

### KEY POINTS
### The Neck

- Neck structures are arranged in bundles which are surrounded by fascia. These have potential spaces between them which may become involved in disease
- In the neck, one or two small, soft, mobile, palpable lymph nodes are quite normal, especially in children
- FNAC is the single most useful primary investigation in diagnosing neck lumps
- Midline swellings are likely to be of thyroid origin if they move on swallowing, or dermoid cysts if they do not
- Neck lumps which could represent a malignancy must be referred to an ENT surgeon in order to search for a primary site
- Subtyping lymphomas usually requires an excisional biopsy in order to study the micro-anatomy of the affected node

**9**

# The ear

**The external ear** 90
Clinical anatomy of the external ear 90
Congenital anomalies 91
Ear wax 91
Otitis externa 92
Trauma to the external ear 93
Neoplastic disorders 95

**The middle ear** 95
Clinical anatomy of the middle ear 95
Symptoms of middle-ear disease 99
Congenital middle-ear conditions 99
Otitis media 100
Cholesteatoma 103
Trauma to the middle ear 106
Neoplastic disorders 106
Otosclerosis 106

**The inner ear** 107
Clinical anatomy of the inner ear 107
The mechanism of hearing 109
Congenital disorders of the inner ear 110
Presbycusis 110
Labyrinthitis 110
Vascular disorders 111
Acoustic trauma 111
Temporal bone trauma 112
Drug ototoxicity 113
Ménière's disease 113
Benign paroxysmal positional vertigo 114
Vestibular neuronitis 114
Acoustic neuromas and CPA tumours 115
Facial nerve 115
Vertigo 117
Tinnitus 118
Hearing loss 118
Assessment of audiological symptoms 119

# THE EXTERNAL EAR

## CLINICAL ANATOMY OF THE EXTERNAL EAR

The external ear is made up of the auricle or pinna and the external auditory meatus. Its function is to collect and transmit sound to the tympanic membrane.

### The auricle

The auricle develops from six nodules or hillocks derived from the first two branchial arches and the overlying skin. The auricle is formed by a skeleton of yellow elastic cartilage covered in skin. The auricle consists of a number of named folds (Figure 9.1).

### The external auditory meatus (EAM)

The external auditory meatus is a tube which connects the conchal bowl to the tympanic membrane. It consists of two parts: the outer one-third is cartilaginous; the inner or medial two-thirds is bony. Overall, the meatus is 24–25 mm long in the adult. The skin of the outer one-third of the meatus is hair-bearing and contains wax and sebaceous glands. These structures are lost in the inner bony meatus where the skin is thin and hair-free.

The two portions of the meatus have slightly different directions (the cartilaginous upward and backward, the bony forward and downward). Thus, when examining the ear, the auricle should be pulled gently upwards

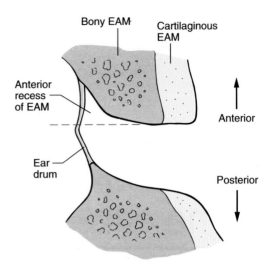

FIGURE 9.2 Horizontal (axial) section through left EAM.

and backwards. This improves the view of the tympanic membrane by straightening the meatus (Figure 9.2).

The nerve supply of the external ear is surprisingly complex. The auriculotemporal branch of the trigeminal nerve supplies most of the anterior half of the auricle and the external auditory meatus. The greater auricular nerve (C2,3), together with branches from the lesser occipital nerve (C2) supply the posterior and the cranial side of the auricle. The IXth and Xth cranial nerves also supply small sensory branches to the ear around the concha, posterior meatus and near the tympanic membrane. It is these branches that when stimulated during examination of the ear (especially in children), can cause an episode of coughing due to vagal stimulation (the recurrent laryngeal nerve is a branch of the vagus). Knowledge of the nerve supply of the ear is important as patients may present with otalgia referred to the ear by stimulation of these nerves elsewhere in their course. A classic example is the otalgia caused by a malignancy in the pyriform fossa of the pharynx (Figure 9.3). Skin cancers which form on this sun-exposed structure may spread via the lymph system to nodes situated either within the parotid gland, to retro-auricular nodes and also to the upper cervical nodes.

The skin of the lateral surface of the tympanic membrane and ear canal is unusual. It is not simply shed as is the skin from the rest of the body, but is migratory and travels radially outwards from the ear drum and thence out along the ear canal. As a result the ears are largely self cleaning (cotton buds simply push wax back down the ear canal). The wax or cerumen which is formed is mildly acidic and has a bacteriostatic effect.

The exposed position of the external ear makes it vulnerable to many disease processes. These can either produce cosmetic abnormalities or affect its function lead-

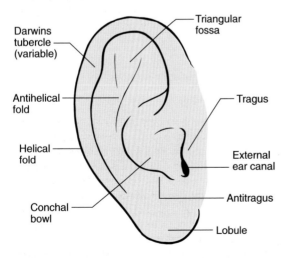

FIGURE 9.1 The auricle consists of a number of named folds.

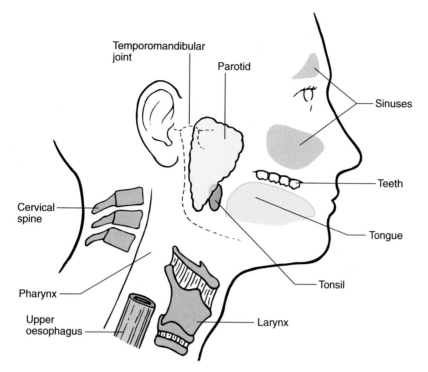

FIGURE 9.3 Causes of referred otalgia.

ing to deafness or tinnitus. The auricle and EAM are both highly sensitive and even mild inflammation, especially in the confined space of the EAM, can lead to pain and the early presentation of the patient to the doctor.

## CONGENITAL ANOMALIES

These can range from total absence of the ear, called anotia, to very mild cosmetic deformities such as tiny accessory auricles or skin tags. External ear anomalies can be isolated or associated with middle- and inner-ear abnormalities, or with the failure of branchial arch development. Here, the combination of abnormalities may present as a syndrome, e.g. Treacher Collins syndrome.

Pre-auricular sinuses are quite common in children. They are due to inadequate fusion of the six hillocks. If they cause symptoms due to infection, they can be excised. Prominent or bat ears are caused by failure of the normal formation of the folds of the auricle. Surgical correction is straightforward.

## EAR WAX

Ear wax (or cerumen), which blocks the EAM, is probably the most common ear problem in the general population. As we have already mentioned, the ear canal will naturally shed wax from the ear. However, in some cases (usually after misguided attempts to clean the ears), wax can completely block the EAM at which point it causes a hearing loss. Further attempts at cleaning the ears lead to trauma and a secondary otitis externa may develop.

Wax-softening agents such as sodium bicarbonate ear drops are the first line of treatment. If this fails, then the ears may be syringed providing there are no contraindications, e.g. tympanic membrane perforation, grommet *in situ*, previous ear surgery or pain which suggests an otitis externa.

Ear syringing involves flushing the ear with warm water in order to wash out any wax or debris. It is most commonly performed by the practice nurse in the GP surgery. If this fails to remove the wax the patient may need to be referred to the ENT department for wax removal by microsuction.

Remember that until all wax has been removed and all the tympanic membrane visualized, assessment of the ears is incomplete.

# OTITIS EXTERNA

## Acute and chronic otitis externa

This is a common, generalized inflammation of the skin of the EAM. It can occur as an acute episode or run a more chronic course. The cause of otitis externa is often multifactorial. General skin conditions such as eczema predispose to infection with an associated allergic response adding to the symptoms. Local factors such as trauma may initiate the condition. The end result is a swollen, narrowed EAM which is itchy and often acutely tender.

The most frequent causes of otitis externa are:

- General causes
   General skin conditions, e.g. eczema, psoriasis
   Generalized skin infections, e.g. impetigo
   Neurodermatitis
- Local causes
   Trauma, e.g. cotton bud, dirty fingernail
   Local infection
      Bacterial: *Pseudomonas, Staphylococcus*
      Fungal: *Candida, Aspergillus*
      Viral
   Middle-ear discharge

A typical course of events may be as follows: bath water is allowed to enter the ear canal and an allergic, eczematous response to the soapy water occurs; this causes itching. Scratching the ear canal with a fingernail or cotton bud causes local trauma and allows a portal of entry for infection and so further inflammation. Itchiness and irritation of the EAM gradually builds up to an ache or pain. Otorrhoea (aural discharge) begins. The skin of the meatus becomes swollen and partly or totally occludes the ear canal which may lead to hearing loss. The inflammation may spread to the auricle causing perichondritis (Figure 9.4) and then to the surrounding tissues, causing facial cellulitis.

*(Remember, the external ear canal does not have any mucous glands. Therefore, if the discharge coming from the ear is mucinous, it must have originated from the **middle** ear and the patient **must** have a perforation in the eardrum with underlying middle-ear infection or cholesteatoma even if this cannot be seen. It must always be borne in mind that otitis externa can develop secondary to this middle-ear suppuration.)*

On examination, the auricle and specifically the tragus, is tender on movement. There may be some

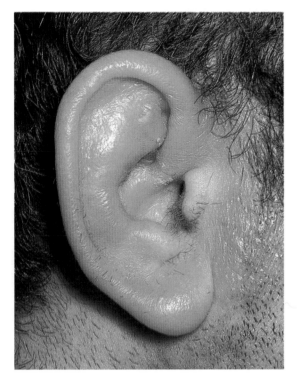

FIGURE 9.4 Perichondritis.

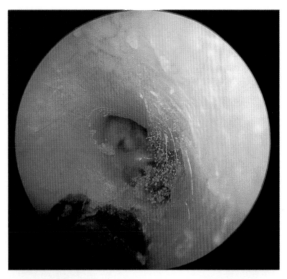

FIGURE 9.5 Fungal otitis externa. Note the fungal hyphae. Published with the kind permission of Mr C. Milford FRCS.

tenderness behind the ear if the lymph nodes there become involved. The EAM becomes swollen and full of debris, sometimes obscuring the tympanic membrane, and the skin can be cracked and crusting. In fungal infections, hyphae and spores can sometimes be seen (Figure 9.5). In chronic otitis externa, the skin of the EAM may be thickened, fissured and permanently moist. Occasionally, a meatal stenosis can develop.

### Treatment

An ear swab should be taken for microbiological examination. The aim of therapy is to remove any irritant factors and treat both infection and any underlying skin disorders.

- Aural toilet: all possible debris is removed from the EAM either with suction and the aid of a microscope or dry mopping.
- Local medication: antibiotic/steroid ear drops:
  antifungal agents
  glycerin and ichthammol
  aluminium acetate
  steroid creams
  These medications can be used as drops or on a wick to pack the EAM.
- Systemic antibiotics for gross cellulitis.

As the EAM inflammation settles, the tympanic membrane must be inspected in order to exclude middle-ear disease as the underlying cause of the condition. The patient should be warned not to let water into the ears (cotton wool smeared with Vaseline can help prevent this) and not to put any object (finger or cotton bud) in their ear. This will also help to prevent recurrent episodes.

### Malignant otitis externa

This condition is poorly named, since it is not in any way neoplastic. It is, however, a lethal condition which must be treated with great respect.

Malignant otitis externa is a more aggressive form of otitis externa, usually seen in the elderly and diabetics. The causative organism is *Pseudomonas*, which spreads to bone, producing an osteitis or osteomyelitis of the skull base. Great pain, granulations in the meatus and cranial nerve palsies are the clinical features. The facial nerve (VIIth) and those exiting from the jugular foramen (IXth, Xth, XIth) can be involved in the infection as it spreads across the skull base. There is a definite mortality rate and treatment needs to be prompt with high-dose intravenous antibiotics and sometimes surgical debridement.

## TRAUMA TO THE EXTERNAL EAR

The position of the auricle on the head and its soft, non-bony structure makes it very vulnerable to trauma from a variety of sources.

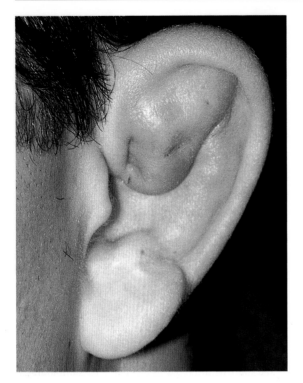

FIGURE 9.6 A traumatic haematoma of the pinna requiring drainage.

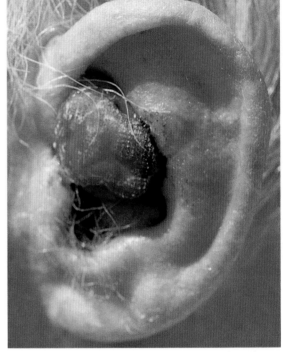

FIGURE 9.7 A squamous cell carcinoma of the pinna.

## Blunt trauma

Blows to the ear can cause bruising. However, in the auricle, blood can track between the perichondrium and the cartilage and a *haematoma auris* results (Figure 9.6). This blood clot can organize, causing dense scarring and thickening of the ear. If infection of the clot occurs, necrosis of the cartilage and gross deformity may follow. This is known as a cauliflower ear. Treatment is by aspiration or incision and drainage, followed by pressure and antibiotic cover (see also Chapter 13, page 161).

## Sharp trauma

This can vary from minor lacerations to complete auricular avulsion. The external ear has a very good blood supply and, as a result, even extensive injuries will often heal well.

## Thermal trauma

The exposed auricle may become frost-bitten in low temperatures. Rewarming is usually successful but debridement of gangrenous tissue may be required.

## Foreign bodies

Beads, stones, nuts and other small objects often find their way into children's ears. Presentation occurs either after the child tells their parent, or if pain, discharge or deafness intervene. In adults cotton wool from 'ear buds' is common. Removal can often be achieved in a cooperative subject, but sometimes a general anaesthetic is needed if the object is near the tympanic membrane. See also Chapter 13, page 158.

### KEY POINTS
Otitis Externa

- Main symptoms include: pain, itch, discharge and hearing loss
- Patients must be told not to scratch the ear, use cotton buds or allow water into the ear
- The mainstay of treatment is aural toilet, with dry mopping or microsuction
- Use topical combination antibiotic and steroid ear drops along with adequate analgesia
- Malignant otitis externa is potentially fatal and affects the elderly, diabetics and the immunocompromised

# NEOPLASTIC DISORDERS

## Benign

Any benign skin neoplasm such as papillomas and adenomas can present in the external ear. Bony exostoses arise from the bony meatus and are usually seen in patients who spend a great deal of time in cold water, e.g. windsurfers or swimmers. They can slowly occlude the meatus leading to failure of wax extrusion and deafness. Treatment of such benign lesions is by local excision (using a drill in the case of exostoses).

## Malignant

Basal cell and squamous cell carcinomas (Figure 9.7) are the commonest tumours of the auricle. Both may present as ulcerating or crusting lesions which grow slowly and may be ignored by older patients. Basal cell carcinomas rarely metastasize and treatment is by complete local excision with skin grafting if necessary, or by radiotherapy. Squamous cell carcinomas may metastasize to the parotid or neck nodes and need aggressive treatment. Wide excision of such lesions on the auricle may be necessary. Carcinomas of the meatus cause pain and, due to their position, involve more radical surgery sometimes with total excision of the external ear and meatus. Metastases spread to the parotid and upper cervical lymph nodes. If this has occurred, radical parotidectomy with or without neck dissection may be required. The use of radiotherapy must also be considered.

## CASE STUDY

Steve is 17-years-old and has just returned from a Spanish holiday. He is complaining of severe right-sided earache with a reduction in his hearing over the last two days. Prior to this, he had complained to his family of intense itching in the ear and had used cotton buds to scratch his ear. In the past he had required ear syringing for wax impaction. He is not diabetic.

1   What is the most likely diagnosis?
2   How should he be treated?
3   What advice should he be given prior to leaving the consultation?
4   Why is it important to review the patient?
5   What is the relevance of diabetes in this condition?

**Comments**
1   Otitis externa.
2   Aural toilet, which may consist in mopping the ear or microsuction, is the mainstay of treatment. Topical combination, antibiotic and steroid ear drops will further speed recovery in the majority of cases. The condition is frequently very painful and adequate analgesia is also necessary.
3   The patient must be told to protect his ears from water and not to put cotton buds or any other object into his ears. He must be instructed in the correct instillation of ear drops and a follow-up appointment made.
4   The patient should be reviewed to ensure the condition has resolved and to allow adequate examination of the ear drum, which is frequently obscured at the first attendance, due to canal oedema. This is necessary since very occasionally otitis externa can be secondary to chronic middle-ear disease such as chronic suppurative otitis media or cholesteatoma.
5   Malignant otitis externa is a potentially fatal, spreading, skull base osteomyelitis which usually occurs in elderly diabetics and must be recognized.

# THE MIDDLE EAR

# CLINICAL ANATOMY OF THE MIDDLE EAR

The middle-ear cleft or tympanic cavity is an air-filled space that is situated within the petrous temporal bone. It is made up of the mastoid air cells, the middle ear itself, the tympanic membrane and eustachian tube. Its function is to transmit sounds, which reach the tympanic membrane in the form of air-pressure waves, to the fluid containing inner ear where a liquid wave is set up. The sound energy is transmitted across the middle ear by a chain of three bones (malleus, incus and stapes) or ossicles. The ossicular chain, together with the ear drum, also amplify the sound energy (Figure 9.8). The middle-ear cleft has the shape of a biconcave disc, rather similar to that of a red blood cell. It is about 1.5 cm in diameter. Posteriorly, it connects via the aditus and antrum to the mastoid air cells. The eustachian tube opens into the anterior part of the middle ear.

The tympanic membrane makes up most of the lateral wall. It consists of three layers: an outer squamous epithelial layer which is in continuity with the

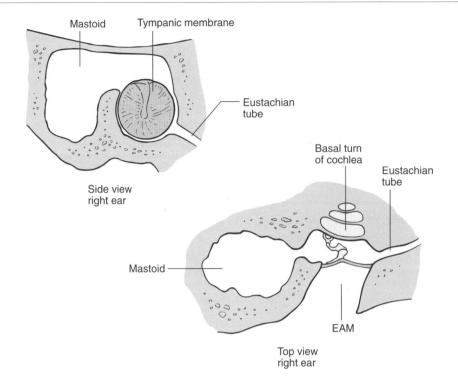

FIGURE 9.8 The middle-ear cleft and mastoid.

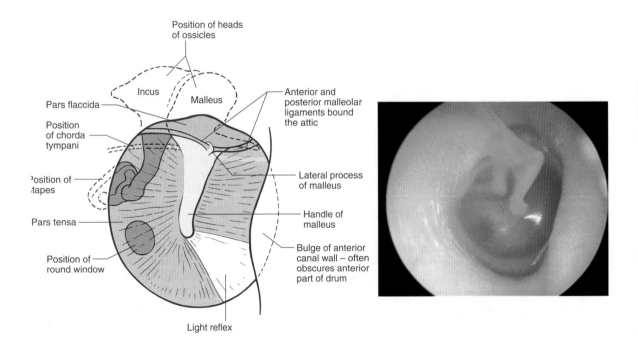

FIGURE 9.9 A normal right ear drum. Otoscopic appearance.

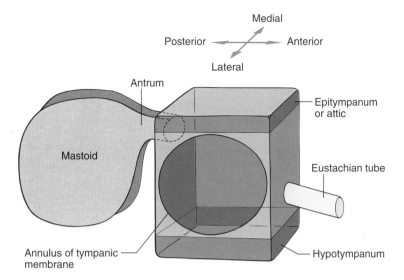

FIGURE 9.10 Schematic diagram of middle-ear cleft and mastoid.

external meatus, a fibrous middle layer and an inner layer continuous with the middle-ear mucosa. It lies obliquely to the meatus and several features are visible on inspection (Figure 9.9).

The handle of the malleus is attached to the tympanic membrane. It is easily seen and used as a reference point when describing abnormalities of the ear drum. The middle fibrous layer radiates out from the malleus. A condensation of this fibrous layer attaches into a bony sulcus in the surrounding bone. This is known as the annulus.

Superiorly (above the anterior and posterior malleolar ligaments) lies a small segment of the tympanic membrane where the fibrous layer is missing; this area is named the pars flaccida, since it is thinner than the remainder of the drum which is named the pars tensa. When light is shone onto the tympanic membrane, it is maximally reflected from the anterio-inferior quadrant; this is because the drum is somewhat cone shaped. A normal tympanic membrane should be pearly grey and slightly translucent. The squamous epithelium of the outermost layer of the tympanic membrane is unusual since it is migratory; it creeps radially outwards away from the handle of the malleus to the edge of the drum and from here moves laterally along the ear canal. This means that debris is also carried out of the ear canal and build up of dead skin does not occur. Defects in the migration of this squamous epithelium can lead to disease, most notably cholesteatoma.

The anatomy of the middle ear may be better understood if it is compared to a box (Figure 9.10).

The *medial wall* of the tympanic cavity has two openings into the inner ear. These are the round and

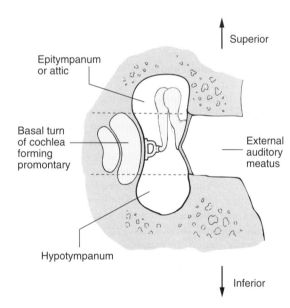

FIGURE 9.11 Transverse section through middle ear.

oval windows and are situated posteriorly in the medial wall. The promontory occupies the central part of the medial wall and is a bulge caused by the basal turn of the cochlea. Its apex lies at the same level as the tip of the handle of the malleus and this is where the middle ear cavity is at its narrowest (Figure 9.11). The facial nerve runs in a bony channel, called the fallopian canal, across the medial wall of the middle ear. It

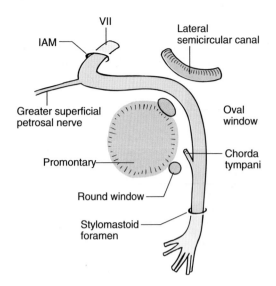

FIGURE 9.12 The medial wall of the middle ear.

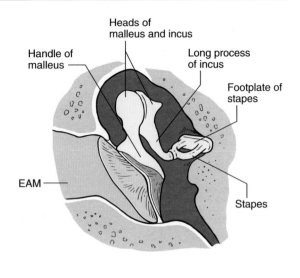

FIGURE 9.13 The ossicles.

courses posteriorly above the oval window, and then turns through 90° below the opening of the aditus of the antrum and descends to exit the base of the skull via the stylomastoid foramen (Figure 9.12).

The anterior wall of the tympanic cavity has two openings: the eustachian tube orifice below and the canal which houses the tensor tympani muscle above. The eustachian tube is part bony and part cartilaginous. It passes medially and forwards to communicate with the nasopharynx. Its function is to allow air to pass freely between the nasal and middle-ear cavities. This not only allows oxygen to reach the mucosa of the middle ear but also ensures similar pressures apply to either side of the eardrum (this is required in order that the tympanic membrane is able to vibrate freely and hence sound transmission to be maximal). Muscles of the pharynx attach to its cartilaginous portion and open the tube when swallowing occurs.

The floor of the middle ear is composed of a plate of bone that lies over the bulb of the jugular vein. This can sometimes be dehiscent and the jugular bulb can be seen as a blue crescent through the tympanic membrane.

There are three ossicles: the malleus, the incus and the stapes (Figure 9.13) which are connected by synovial joints. The stapes is the smallest of the ossicles; its footplate occupies the oval window. Vibrations here set up a fluid wave in the liquid-filled inner ear which lies under the stapes footplate. In this way, an air-pressure wave is converted to a liquid one and it is this which stimulates the cochlea, the organ of hearing.

The ossicles transmit sound from the tympanic membrane to the oval window but they also allow amplification. This is achieved by two mechanisms. Firstly, there is a 14:1 ratio between the size of the

tympanic membrane and that of the oval window. Secondly, there is a gain due to the lever action of the ossicles themselves. Altogether there is an 18:1 amplification in sound pressure simply due to the mechanics of the middle ear.

Infection of the middle ear, or otitis media, is common. Spread of infection beyond the middle ear can occur and can affect any of its relations.

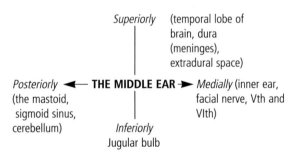

### KEY POINTS
Anatomy of the Middle Ear

- The ossicles transmit sound across the middle ear
- The pars flaccida is thin and more susceptible to pressure changes within the middle ear
- The outer layer of the tympanic membrane consists of squamous epithelium and migrates out of the ear along the ear canal
- The facial nerve runs through the middle ear
- The eustachian tube allows air to enter the middle-ear cavity

## OVERVIEW
### Diseases of the Middle Ear

**Congenital**
- Agenesis of the middle ear cleft: may be associated with external/inner-ear anomalies
- Ossicular abnormality/fixation
- Round/oval window agenesis
- Facial nerve dehiscence/abnormal path
- **Cholesteatoma**

**Infective/inflammatory**
- **Glue ear = otitis media with effusion = secretory otitis media**
- **Acute suppurative otitis media**
- **Chronic suppurative otitis media**
- **Cholesteatoma**
- **Otosclerosis**
- Tuberculous otitis media
- Granulomatous disorders, e.g. Wegener's granulomatosis

**Traumatic**
- **Tympanic membrane perforation**
- Ossicular dislocation
- Temporal bone fractures
- Barotrauma

**Neoplastic**
- Benign
  - Adenoma
  - Osteoma
  - Meningioma
  - Neurogenic
  - Glomus tumours
- Malignant
  - Squamous carcinoma
  - Adenocarcinoma

# SYMPTOMS OF MIDDLE-EAR DISEASE

Many conditions which affect the middle ear present with broadly similar symptoms.

## Hearing loss

This is of the conductive type and is easily demonstrable with tuning fork testing (Rinne's BC > AC and Weber localizes to the affected side).

## Tinnitus

This symptom can occur in association with a hearing loss of any cause, but if pulsatile, should arouse suspicion of a vascular tumour close to the ear.

## Pain (otalgia)

This is most commonly due to a rapidly accumulating effusion in the middle ear such as occurs in acute otitis media. Here, the eardrum becomes stretched, causing intense pain. Once the drum perforates, the pressure is released and the pain resolves. Carcinoma and Wegener's granulomatosis also cause deep-seated otalgia.

## Ear discharge (otorrhoea)

This is usually due to infection of the middle mucosa and results in a mucopurulent discharge. This may also fill the ear canal if there is a hole in the drum. Infection can spread to structures closely related to the middle ear and it is very important that one asks about symptoms such as vertigo, facial nerve weakness and headache.

# CONGENITAL MIDDLE-EAR CONDITIONS

Congenital anomalies of the middle ear may be isolated or associated with other ear or general congenital deformities. There is a number of paediatric syndromes where external and middle-ear abnormalities are common. Examples include first branchial arch syndromes such as Pierre–Robin, craniofacial dysostosis, Down's syndrome and Treacher Collins syndrome. The presence of any external ear abnormality must always raise the suspicion of underlying middle-ear deformity but remember the *inner* ear in such cases can be normal as it develops via a different pathway to the external and middle ear. Hence, reconstruction of the conducting system or bone-conducting hearing aid can achieve a good hearing threshold.

Congenital disorders of the middle ear may be suspected due to external ear or other associated abnormalities, or may be recognized by the failure of the child to react to noise. Sometimes mild anomalies may only present in later life with a slight hearing loss. Full assessment with radiology of the temporal bones is essential. If the inner ear appears normal, surgical reconstruction of the middle ear can be very success-

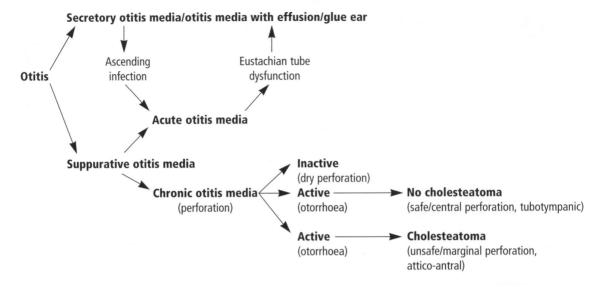

ful. Cochlear implantation or a hearing aid should also be considered in some cases.

# OTITIS MEDIA

Inflammation of the middle ear is characterized by the formation of an effusion. This can either be sterile (as in glue ear) or may occur as a result of suppurative (pus-forming) infection (as in acute otitis media). Repeated attacks of acute suppuration can lead to weakening of the eardrum and eventually to a non-healing perforation. This is now chronic suppurative otitis media (CSOM). CSOM has been classified into different types depending on the position of the perforation within the drum. One classification uses the terms 'tubotympanic' and 'attico-antral', another 'central' and 'marginal'. As a result of these classifications, attempts have been made to predict the likelihood of the patient developing a cholesteatoma and the terms *safe* and *unsafe* refer to this risk. We find these terms at best confusing and prefer to state if there is active infection (i.e. otorrhoea) or not, and moreover, to state if a cholesteatoma is present or not, since both otorrhoea and cholesteatoma are usually evident on simple examination.

## Acute otitis media (Figure 9.14)

This acute infection of the middle-ear cleft is common in children and is usually associated with an upper respiratory tract infection which spreads to the middle ear via the eustachian tube. An accumulation of pus within the middle ear leads to pressure on the tym-

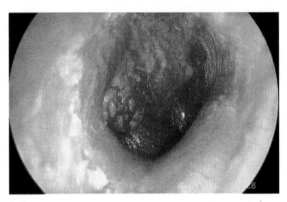

FIGURE 9.14 Acute otitis media of the right ear; note the bulging, inflamed, red drum.

panic membrane, and hence pain. Rupture of the tympanic membrane with otorrhoea and a rapid reduction in otalgia may follow. The symptoms are:

- Hearing loss
- Pain
- Otorrhoea
- Pyrexia
- Systemic upset

It should be remembered that small children may give few, if any, localizing signs and may simply present with pyrexia and systemic upset. In all such cases, a thorough ENT examination must be performed.

As the infection abates, mucosal oedema subsides, the effusion slowly resolves and any tympanic membrane perforation heals. In many young children, this becomes a recurring problem, probably as a result of repeated reinfection of the pool of stagnant glue filling the middle ear. If a six-week course of low-dose antibiotics fails to break this cycle of infections, grommet insertion may be considered, even if the hearing remains satisfactory. The causative agents may be either viral or bacterial, but *Haemophilus influenzae* or *Streptococcus pneumoniae* are most common.

Treatment is with antibiotics such as amoxycillin and simple analgesia. If there is a perforation, the ear must be kept dry until it has healed. In a discharging ear, combination antibiotic and steroid ear drops can also be used. Nasal decongestants may speed recovery by improving eustachian tube function and hence middle-ear ventilation. Most episodes of otitis media resolve completely. However, damage to the ear can occur. For example:

- Residual perforation
- Residual effusion
- Necrosis of the ossicles.
- Tympanosclerosis – white scarring of the tympanic membrane
- Ossicular adhesions

If the infection spreads beyond the middle-ear cleft, serious complications can occur.

## Otitis media with effusion (glue ear)
### (Figure 9.15)

This condition has been given many names: secretory otitis media (SOM), non-suppurative otitis media, otitis media with effusion (OME), or more commonly 'glue ear'. The underlying basis of the disorder is poor ventilation of the middle ear cavity which leads to a sterile (non-purulent) and often thick and sticky effusion. A number of factors may have a role to play in this condition but the exact cause remains uncertain. Some possible causes include:

- A sequelae of acute otitis media
- Infection or allergy of the middle-ear mucosa
- Eustachian tube dysfunction resulting from:
  poor/delayed development
  obstruction due to large adenoid
  nasal abnormalities/conditions
  cleft palate

Glue ear affects 70–80% of children at some time in their lives. In most, it resolves spontaneously. However, in a small, but significant, number it can last months or years. The main effect of glue ear is upon the hearing. It usually leads to a mild loss with a reduction of between 20 and 30 dB in the hearing threshold. In the long term, hearing loss can disrupt the child's behaviour and schooling. A chronic effusion can also predispose to repeated attacks of acute otitis media as a result of infection spreading to the fluid-filled middle ear via the eustachian tube.

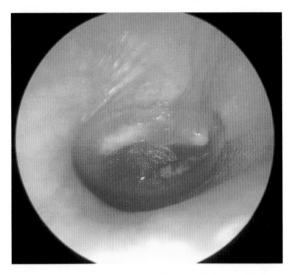

FIGURE 9.15 Glue ear. Note the dullness and slight yellow tinge to the drum. Also the radial blood vessels and more horizontally placed malleus handle. The light reflex is absent.

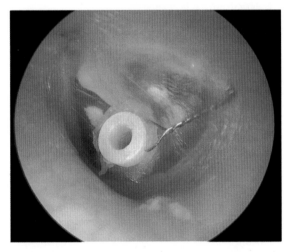

FIGURE 9.16 A grommet (with wire) placed in the right ear drum.

If the glue does not resolve over three months, and if it is symptomatic, treatment may be required. Currently, the main treatment consists of the insertion of grommets. These are small plastic tubes that are inserted into the tympanic membrane and remain there for usually one to two years before being slowly extruded (Figure 9.16). They provide an alternative route for middle ear ventilation; hence the effusion resolves, and as a result, the hearing returns to normal. Most children grow out of their glue ear and so it is hoped that by the time the grommets extrude, the eustachian tube will function normally and so the glue will not return. However, occasionally a child may need repeated insertions of grommets if the effusion re-accumulates. Hearing aids boost the hearing and are an alternative to grommets in some cases.

## CASE STUDY

Simon is four years old and his mother is worried that he does not hear as well as his six-year-old sister. She has also been told by the teachers at his playgroup that he is often naughty and ignores them. They also find it difficult to understand him. He has had more than his fair share of ear infections and snores most nights. His mother has noted that his snoring is worse when he has a cold and on occasions she has been worried about his breathing at night. On examination he appears well today, but is breathing through his mouth. He has massive tonsils, but has not suffered with tonsillitis, and his eardrums appear dull and a little retracted.

1  What is the most likely cause of his hearing loss and how should this be investigated?
2  Apart from his hearing loss, what else concerns you about this young boy?
3  Outline how you think he should be treated.

### Comments

1  It is most likely that this boy has glue ear, not only because it is the most common cause of hearing problems in children, but also because of the appearances on otoscopy and the fact that he has nasal symptoms which are consistent with adenoid hypertrophy. A hearing assessment and tympanometry should be performed.
2  His poor speech development and apparent poor performance at school are of some concern. Recurrent ear infections are also associated with glue ear. Snoring and problems breathing at night are suggestive of the obstructive sleep apnoea syndrome. Other indications in this case are his poor behaviour and concentration at school and poor nasal airway.
3  In the first instance, a short period of watchful waiting may be appropriate in order to ensure that he is not about to grow out of his problems. If after three months he is no better, most ENT surgeons would offer him adenoidectomy and grommet insertion to treat his glue ear and nasal symptoms, as well as tonsillectomy in view of the history suggestive of obstructive sleep apnoea.

## Chronic suppurative otitis media (CSOM)

Repeated or prolonged bouts of acute otitis media, often in childhood, can cause damage to the tympanic membrane and a non-healing perforation may result. The perforation may occupy either the pars flaccida or the pars tensa. Perforations may also be further described as central or marginal, depending on their position relative to the annulus of the drum (Figures

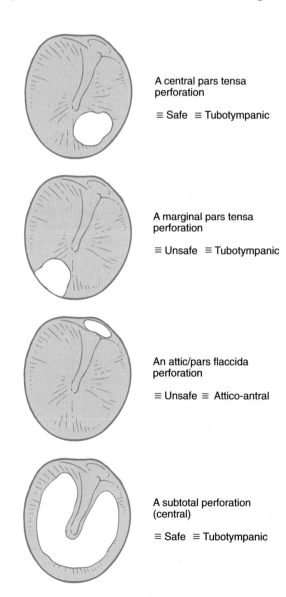

A central pars tensa perforation

≡ Safe  ≡ Tubotympanic

A marginal pars tensa perforation

≡ Unsafe  ≡ Tubotympanic

An attic/pars flaccida perforation

≡ Unsafe  ≡ Attico-antral

A subtotal perforation (central)

≡ Safe  ≡ Tubotympanic

FIGURE 9.17 Types of tympanic membrane perforation.

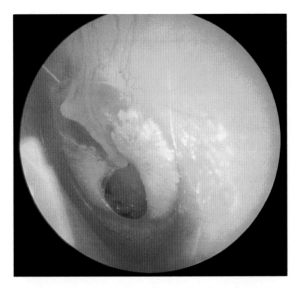

FIGURE 9.18 An inferiorly placed, central, safe perforation. Note the marked tympanosclerosis of the drum indicating previous inflammation.

9.17 and Figure 9.18). Chronic infection of the middle ear may often spread to involve the mastoid system, and the infected mucosa of these areas produces copious amounts of mucopus, which leaks through the tympanic membrane perforation into the external ear canal. This can sometimes be mistaken for otitis externa if the perforation is obscured by discharge. As the infection is overcome, either naturally or with treatment, the ear becomes dry (inactive CSOM) and the perforation will be seen. CSOM often runs an intermittent course with bouts of discharge (active CSOM), occurring either as a result of simple upper respiratory tract infections spreading up the eustachian tube or from water entering the EAM and hence to the middle ear via the tympanic membrane perforation.

## Symptoms

The symptoms of CSOM are:

■ Hearing loss
■ Otorrhoea
  intermittent
  mucoid/mucopurulent

The hearing loss is usually mild (10–20 dB) if only the tympanic membrane is involved; in some cases, the ossicular chain can become damaged. The most usual site of ossicular disruption is the long process of the incus, since this has the most tenuous blood supply and in this case the hearing loss is more severe (50–70 dB).

## Treatment

Treatment depends on the symptoms. Regular aural toilet plus combination antibiotic and steroid ear drops, and keeping the ear dry, will help to settle active infection. Surgical repair of the eardrum (myringoplasty), if successful, will prevent reinfection. Some patients with inactive CSOM have few if any symptoms, and in these no treatment is required.

Active CSOM can occasionally be complicated by spread of the infection to other structures in just the same way as in acute otitis media.

# CHOLESTEATOMA

Cholesteatoma is a poor name since this condition is not a tumour, as the suffix '-oma' may suggest. Also, it has nothing what so ever to do with cholesterol! A cholesteatoma is, in fact, a cyst, or sac of keratinizing squamous epithelium (skin) and most commonly occurs in the attic or epitympanic part of the middle ear. Frequently, a cholesteatoma will cause a chronic, foul-smelling discharge, and as a result is classified as a sub-type of CSOM known as CSOM with cholesteatoma.

The symptoms and signs of cholesteatoma are:

■ Foul-smelling discharge
■ Conductive hearing loss
■ Attic retraction filled with squamous debris
■ Discharging attic perforation
■ Attic aural polyp

Patients may present solely with a complication of cholesteatoma, for example:

■ Facial palsy
■ Vertigo
■ Intracranial sepsis

Cholesteatomas are rarely congenital, and these are thought to arise from 'squamous rest cells' within the middle ear. In the more common, acquired form of the disease, the exact aetiology is unknown. However, the most commonly held view is that negative pressure within the middle ear has a maximal effect on the thin pars flaccida of the tympanic membrane. This has the effect of causing it, or part of it, to balloon backwards forming a so-called 'retraction pocket'. The migratory epithelium of the outer layer of the tympanic membrane may now 'fall' into this pocket and in some cases cannot escape (Figure 9.19 and Figure 9.20). This ball of squamous debris slowly enlarges and invariably becomes infected with *Pseudomonas*, hence the foul otorrhoea. It tends to grow upwards into the attic and backwards into the mastoid. Cholesteatoma is able to erode bone and therefore can damage any of

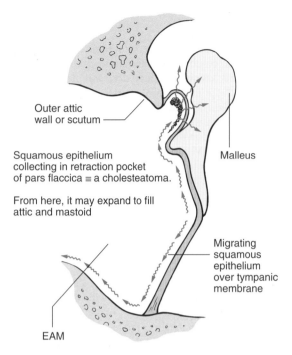

FIGURE 9.19 A schematic diagram to show the formation of a cholesteatoma.

Outer attic wall or scutum

Squamous epithelium collecting in retraction pocket of pars flaccica ≡ a cholesteatoma.

From here, it may expand to fill attic and mastoid

Malleus

Migrating squamous epithelium over tympanic membrane

EAM

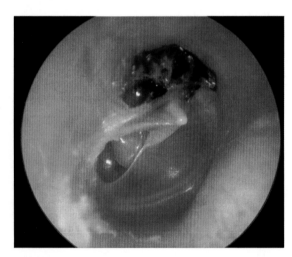

FIGURE 9.20 A cholesteatoma.

## CASE STUDY

John is 24 years old and has had problems with his ears for most of his life. He has had three sets of grommets for glue ear and had numerous ear infections. However, now he has had a constant discharge from his right ear for the last three months. Although this does not bother him greatly, his girlfriend has urged him to see a doctor because of the offensive smell coming from his ear recently. Examination shows the ear canal to be full of debris and mucus, and once this had been removed, a polyp was seen to be filling most of the ear canal, obscuring the tympanic membrane.

1  What is the most likely diagnosis?
2  What other points should be noted on examination?
3  How should he be investigated?

**Comments**

1  Cholesteatomas of the ear frequently present with *offensive*, unilateral otorrhoea. His history of previous ear problems is also suggestive that he may be at some increased risk of developing a cholesteatoma. The other less-worrying diagnosis is active chronic suppurative otitis media (CSOM) without cholesteatoma. In this case, the tympanic membrane would be perforated, and the middle-ear cleft infected, with polyp formation if severe.
2  Examination of the facial nerve is essential, as is testing for nystagmus and performing the fistula test. Tuning fork testing will confirm the presence of a conductive hearing loss on the right side.
3  An audiogram will confirm the conductive hearing loss. The diagnosis of cholesteatoma is clinical and scanning the ear is not necessary unless there is a complication such as a facial nerve palsy. In some cases, it may be necessary to examine the ear under general anaesthesia in order to confirm the diagnosis.

the important structures in or around the middle ear and mastoid, for example:

■ Ossicles – leading to a conductive deafness
■ Facial nerve – and hence facial palsy
■ Labyrinth – leading to vertigo
■ Erosion of the tegmen (roof of the middle ear) leading to intracranial sepsis

Treatment of a cholesteatoma requires surgical removal. The operation required depends on the size and extent of the disease. A small cholesteatoma limited to the attic may only require an 'atticotomy'. More advanced disease which extends into the mastoid will frequently require a 'modified radical mastoidectomy' (Figure 9.21).

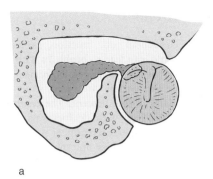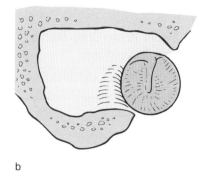

a                                                            b

FIGURE 9.21 (a) An attic cholesteatoma extending backwards into the mastoid. (b) Modified radical mastoidectomy. Here the cholesteatoma has been removed and the mastoid cavity 'exteriorized', i.e. connected to the ear canal by removal of the posterior ear canal wall.

## Complications of otitis media

Complications occur when the infection spreads outside the middle ear. This can occur due to the involvement or erosion of bone, or when there is thrombophlebitis of communicating blood vessels which transmit infection. Fewer complications are seen nowadays due to antibiotic usage. However, when they do occur, they must be recognized since they are serious and may be potentially fatal. They can be divided into extra- and intracranial.

### Extracranial complications

#### Mastoiditis

The mastoid air cells fill with pus. Erosion of bone can lead to swelling behind the ear and thickening of the postauricular tissues which leads to the pinna becoming pushed out (Figure 9.22). A subperiosteal abscess may form behind the ear when infection has broken through the bone.

#### Facial nerve palsy

This is due to inflammation and swelling of the VIIth nerve in its bony canal.

#### Labyrinthitis

This is spread of infection to the inner ear and will cause severe vertigo.

#### Petrositis

This is spread of infection to the petrous bone and can involve the Vth and VIth cranial nerves.

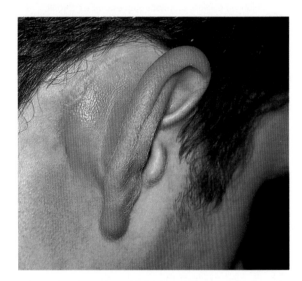

FIGURE 9.22 Mastoiditis: thickening of the postauricular tissues pushes the ear out and makes it look more prominent.

### Intracranial complications

These are:

- Temporal lobe abscess
- Cerebellar abscess
- Sigmoid sinus thrombosis
- Meningitis
- Jugular vein thrombosis
- Otitic hydrocephalus

## KEY POINTS
### Secretory Otitis Media, Acute Otitis Media, Chronic Suppurative Otitis Media, Cholesteatoma

- Glue ear (secretory otitis media) is common in children and often leads to a mild hearing loss
- Abnormal eustachian tube function and poor middle-ear ventilation are believed to cause glue ear
- Prolonged, symptomatic glue ear is most often treated by grommet insertion
- Acute otitis media is common and usually mild and self-limiting
- Complications of acute otitis media, although rare, may be serious and even fatal
- Prolonged painless otorrhoea suggests either chronic suppurative otitis media or cholesteatoma
- Otorrhoea should initially be treated with a short course of combination antibiotic and steroid ear drops
- Foul-smelling ear discharge often accompanies a cholesteatoma

# TRAUMA TO THE MIDDLE EAR

The tympanic membrane and ossicles can be injured either directly or indirectly. Some of the common causes are as follows:

- *Foreign body.* Any object that can fit into the meatus may injure the tympanic membrane. Cotton buds used to clean the ears are the most common offending instrument. Tympanic membrane perforation as well as ossicular disruption can occur with subsequent hearing loss.
- *Air pressure.* A loud explosion, noise or slap to the ear may cause an air-pressure wave forceful enough to cause a perforation or ossicular damage.
- *Head injury.* This may cause a temporal bone fracture with disruption of the bony EAM and drum or can cause ossicular dislocation, even without fracture.

These injuries can cause pain, hearing loss, tinnitus and vertigo. If a traumatic perforation has occurred, the hearing loss is usually of the order of 10–20 dB. If there has been ossicular disruption, the loss will be more in the region of 60 dB. Traumatic perforations often heal, providing the ear is kept clean and dry. Ossicular dislocation demands surgical exploration with re-establishment of ossicular continuity.

## Barotrauma

Poor eustachian tube function, as may occur with a simple cold, can lead to problems with equalizing pressures across the tympanic membrane. Especially when pressure fluctuations are rapid, as in diving or flying particularly during descent. The result may be a middle-ear effusion, with deafness, pain and sometimes vertigo and tinnitus. Treatment is with nasal decongestants, but if this does not succeed, myringotomy and even the insertion of grommets may be necessary.

# NEOPLASTIC DISORDERS

Tumours of the middle ear are rare. The most common of these are squamous cell carcinoma and glomus tumours.

## Squamous cell carcinoma

This usually presents with blood-stained discharge and deep-seated pain. Facial nerve palsy and other signs of infiltration of the tumour occur later. A granular polyp filling the meatus is often found on examination. Squamous carcinomas usually arise in a chronically discharging ear. It is important to note that in all ears with pain and/or bloody otorrhoea, any polyp should be removed and sent for histology. The prognosis, when treated surgically or with radiotherapy, is poor.

## Glomus tumours

These tumours are derived from the paraganglionic cells of nerves around the jugular bulb and may extend into the middle ear. They can cause local destruction by gradual growth and are very vascular. They present classically with pulsatile tinnitus and conductive deafness. In larger tumours the cranial nerves exiting from the jugular foramen may be involved (IXth, Xth and XIth) and pain may also be a feature. Examination of the tympanic membrane may reveal a red mass behind the drum arising from the floor of the middle ear, the so-called 'rising sun' sign. Treatment may simply be observation if the tumour is small since they are very slow growing. Radiotherapy and surgical excision may be required in the larger tumours.

# OTOSCLEROSIS

Otosclerosis is a disease of the otic capsule or bony labyrinth causing hearing loss. The hard, compact

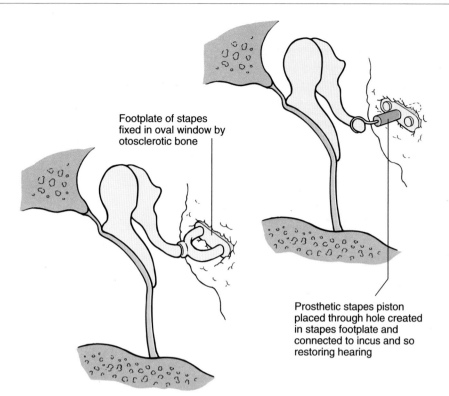

Footplate of stapes
fixed in oval window by
otosclerotic bone

Prosthetic stapes piston
placed through hole created
in stapes footplate and
connected to incus and so
restoring hearing

FIGURE 9.23 The stapedectomy operation.

bone of the labyrinth is replaced by patches of spongy bone, hence the French name *otospongiose*. This abnormal bone is thought to produce toxins which can affect the cochlea causing a sensorineural hearing loss. However, more commonly the bony overgrowth affects the footplate of the stapes, which results in its fixation, and this leads to a conductive hearing loss. The aetiology is unknown but there is an increased incidence in relatives of affected patients. Up to 1 in 100 people may be affected but only a minor proportion of these are symptomatic.

The hearing loss in otosclerosis is predominantly conductive but there may be a sensorineural component as well. It is usually bilateral and begins around the age of 30. Symptoms in women become worse during pregnancy. A number of patients are said to exhibit an unusual symptom called paracusis willsii, i.e. they can hear better when they are in a noisy environment. Tinnitus may be a troublesome feature and occasionally positional vertigo may occur.

The diagnosis should be considered in any patient who presents with a progressive conductive hearing loss and has a normal ear drum. The only way to confirm the diagnosis is by surgical exploration of the middle ear and examination of the stapes footplate. The most common differential diagnosis is ossicular adhesions/fixation.

Treatment may be simply observation if mild, or a hearing aid if symptomatic. A large conductive loss can be treated surgically with an operation called stapedectomy. Here the fixed stapes is removed and replaced by a Teflon piston (Figure 9.23). This can give dramatic results, often with complete return in hearing.

## THE INNER EAR

## CLINICAL ANATOMY OF THE INNER EAR

The inner ear is responsible for both hearing and balance. It consists of a membranous and a bony *labyrinth* (greek = 'maze of tunnels'). The membranous labyrinth consists of a complex system of channels and is surrounded by the rock-hard bony labyrinth. The whole system lies within the petrous part of the temporal bone.

The membranous labyrinth consists of the cochlea, which is responsible for hearing, along with the saccule, utricle and semicircular canals. The latter three

## CASE STUDY

A 33-year-old mother of two complains of poor hearing in the right ear which has become worse during the last year. She admits to some associated tinnitus in the affected ear, but this does not concern her greatly. Examination reveals normal eardrums and tuning fork testing shows a Weber localizing to the right and a negative Rinne test on that side.

1  What is the most likely diagnosis?
2  What other features would you enquire after in order to support your clinical diagnosis?
3  What investigations could you order to support your diagnosis?
4  How may she be treated?

### Comments

1  The tuning fork test suggests a conductive loss and in a young woman with a normal eardrum, the most likely diagnosis is otosclerosis.
2  One should ascertain if there is any family history of deafness, which is found in 60% of patients with otosclerosis. Hearing loss beginning, or worsening, during pregnancy is also suggestive of this diagnosis. Some patients with otosclerosis find that it is easier to hear in noisy environments, although this is not a universal feature. Has there been any balance disturbance associated with her hearing loss?
3  A pure tone audiogram will confirm the conductive hearing loss, and a dip in the bone conduction threshold at 2 kHz (Carhart's notch) is also highly suggestive of otosclerosis. Some specialists order stapedial reflexes, which will be reduced or absent in otosclerosis, in order to confirm the diagnosis.
4  Before any surgical intervention, she should be offered a trial of a hearing aid, since this carries no risk and a proportion of patients will be satisfied with the hearing they achieve. If she does not find a hearing aid suits her, then she may be offered a stapedectomy operation. However, not before she has had all the potential risks of surgery explained to her, not least the fact that occasionally patients who suffer with tinnitus and otosclerosis find the noise gets worse after such an operation.

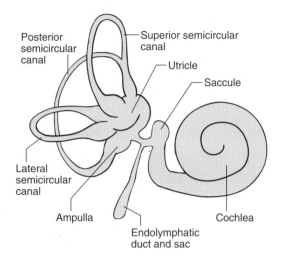

FIGURE 9.24 Membranous labyrinth of the inner ear.

are jointly termed the *vestibular system* and are responsible for balance (Figure 9.24). The bony labyrinth encases and protects these delicate structures. It has a similar shape, other than the utricle and saccule which are together housed in the bony vestibule. The oval and round windows are defects in the bone of the vestibule which in life are closed by the stapes footplate and a membrane respectively.

The membranous labyrinth is filled with a fluid called endolymph. This is similar in composition to an ultrafiltrate of blood (i.e. rich in potassium and deficient in sodium). The membranous labyrinth is itself surrounded by a fluid called perilymph. Perilymph fills the bony labyrinth and has high sodium and low potassium content rather like cerebrospinal fluid (CSF). Although there is a connection between the perilymph and CSF, by means of the cochlear aqueduct, it is not known whether perilymph is totally derived from CSF.

## The vestibular system

There are three semicircular canals named the lateral, superior and posterior. Each lies in a separate plane and communicate via the utricle. Each semicircular canal has a dilation at one end called the ampulla. It is here that the specialized neuroepithelium, which is capable of sensing movement, is situated. There is a similar area of neuroepithelium in the utricle and saccule. These sensory areas consist of hair cells embedded into a thick matrix. The utricle and saccule hair cells are in contact with small particles called otoliths. The area as a whole is known as the macula.

These sensory organs are suspended in the endolymph. When the head moves, the endolymph,

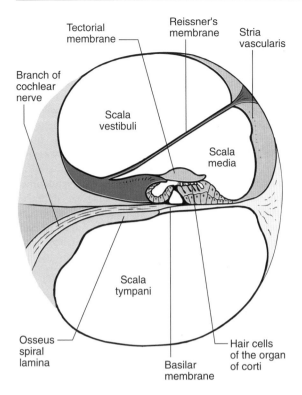

FIGURE 9.25 The cochlea in cross section.

which has its own inertia, takes longer to accelerate than the surrounding labyrinth and neuroepithelium. This leads to a shearing movement of the hair cells or a change in position of the otoliths which stimulates the vestibular nerve appropriately. In this way, movement is detected. The semicircular canals detect rotatory movement, while the saccule and utricle are stimulated by horizontal and vertical acceleration.

## The cochlea

The bony cochlea (Latin = 'snail shell') is a hollow tube, in the form of a spiral, wound with two-and-a-half turns around a central hub, named the modiolus. It is likened to a snail's shell and this is a good analogy. A bony shelf, called the osseous spiral lamina, projects from the central hub into the tube. Two membranes, called Reissner's and the basilar membranes, divide the cochlea into three spaces, the scala media, tympani and scala vestibuli (Figure 9.25).

The scala media or cochlear duct contains endolymph and is linked to the saccule. The scala tympani and vestibuli contain perilymph and communicate with one another at the apex of the cochlea. The sensory unit of the cochlea is called the organ of Corti, and lies on the basilar membrane. It is a complex

structure also composed of hair cells. These hairs are associated with the tectorial membrane that arises from the osseous spiral lamina. The VIIIth nerve endings that supply the hair cells, descend down the modiolus before perforating the base of the cochlea.

## THE MECHANISM OF HEARING

Sound is produced by the vibration of molecules within the air in the form of pressure waves. The ear converts these pressure waves into neural action potentials which are perceived by the brain and central nervous system as hearing. Sound is collected and transmitted to the tympanic membrane by the external ear. These changes in air pressure cause the tympanic membrane to vibrate and, as described in the previous section, they are converted by the ossicles into a rocking motion of the stapes (having been amplified around 18 times).

The stapes footplate overlies the oval window and its movement sets up a pressure wave in the perilymph of the scala vestibuli. The scala vestibuli communicates with the scala tympani and so the perilymph wave travels along the length of these channels and ends at the round window. Since the water-based perilymph is incompressible, movement at the oval window is reciprocated by the opposite movement at the round window (Figure 9.26)

Movement in the perilymph causes vibration of the basilar and the tectorial membranes. The membranes move in a slightly different way to one another and this causes shearing of the hair cells of the organ of Corti. This shearing effect causes stimulation of the hair cells and hence the cochlear nerve. When this impulse reaches the auditory centre of the cortex, sound is perceived. The greater the sound, the larger the perilymph pressure wave and the more the hair cells are stimulated. Different frequencies are detected by differing areas of the cochlea. High frequencies

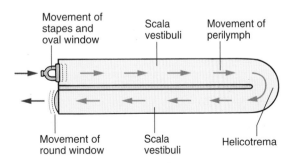

FIGURE 9.26 Diagrammatic representation of perilymph movement in the cochlea (longitudinal section).

stimulate the basal turn, whilst low ones are detected at the cochlear apex.

Inner-ear disease usually presents with sensorineural deafness, tinnitus, vertigo or with a combination of these symptoms. However, one must always consider the possibility of middle-ear disease since this will present with broadly similar symptoms. Remember that pain and ear discharge are not usually features of inner-ear pathology and tend to indicate a middle-ear problem.

---

**OVERVIEW**

**Diseases of the Inner Ear**

**Congenital**
- Labyrinthine aplasia and dysplasia associated with syndromes, e.g. Alport and Waardenburg syndromes
- Intrauterine infection
- **Perinatal labyrinthine damage, e.g. anoxia**

**Acquired**

**Degenerative**
- **Presbycusis**
- **Ménière's disease**

**Infective/inflammatory**
- **Labyrinthitis:** viral, bacterial, syphilis
- Spread from otitis media/cholesteatoma
- Other infections, e.g. mumps

**Vascular**
- **Vascular occlusion**
- Vasculitis, e.g. polyarteritis nodosa, Wegener's granulomatosis

**Traumatic**
- **Acoustic: acute/chronic**
- Direct/labyrinthine concussion
- Temporal bone fractures
- Round/oval window rupture
- **Drug ototoxicity:** gentamicin, etc.
- **Surgical**

**Metabolic**
- Diabetes mellitus
- Thyroid disease

**Other**
- **Otosclerosis**
- **Benign paroxysmal positional vertigo**

---

# CONGENITAL DISORDERS OF THE INNER EAR

Congenital or hereditary inner-ear disorders present with deafness. They may be associated with external or middle-ear abnormalities or exist on their own. The most common anomaly is dysplasia of the membranous labyrinth, although dysplasias of the bony labyrinth and rarely, total aplasia of both may occur. Such deafness can be associated with other clinical anomalies and together comprise a syndrome. Intrauterine infections can cause inner-ear damage. Rubella is the best known, although there are many others. Perinatal hypoxia or anoxia, and Rhesus incompatibility are also risk factors for hearing loss.

# PRESBYCUSIS

Presbycusis, a degenerative disorder, is the term used to describe the hearing loss of old age. This is a common problem in many elderly patients. It is characterized by a gradual hearing loss in both ears with or without tinnitus. Such a hearing loss usually affects the higher frequencies and the audiogram is classical (Figure 9.27). Poor hearing can make communication difficult and tinnitus can also be most distressing to some patients. There is no cure, but a hearing aid can be of great help by amplifying sound and masking the tinnitus. Atrophy of the labyrinth and cochlear nerve fibres cause this condition.

# LABYRINTHITIS

Labyrinthitis is an acute inflammation of the inner ear which usually follows a simple upper respiratory tract infection. However, infection may spread to involve the labyrinth either from middle-ear infection, from intracranial sepsis or via the bloodstream. Vertigo is the most pronounced symptom and may be disabling. It can last for some days, or even weeks, before beginning to settle. There may be some residual vertigo occurring with rapid movements for some months after the initial episode. If the condition is severe, hearing loss may occur, and it can even lead to total vestibular destruction, a so-called 'dead' labyrinth. Treatment is with antibiotics, vestibular sedatives, such as prochlorperazine, and rest. Generally, there is gradual labyrinthine compensation, and this process of rehabilitation may be accelerated with special Cooksey – Cawthorne exercises.

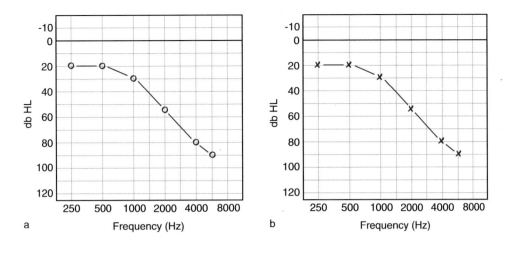

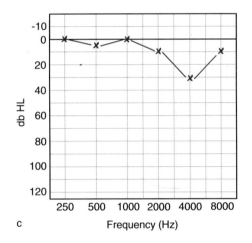

FIGURE 9.27 (a) and (b) Classical audiogram showing hearing loss of old age. (c) Audiogram showing noise-induced hearing loss.

# VASCULAR DISORDERS

Occlusion of, or reduction in, labyrinthine blood flow will lead to hypoxia and inner-ear cell damage. This may be acute, as in thrombosis or embolism, or chronic due to atherosclerosis. Vasculitic diseases such as Wegener's granulomatosis may also give rise to similar changes. Any interruption to the blood supply of the inner ear can lead to hearing loss, with or without tinnitus, and in the acute situation vertigo may also be a prominent feature. Sudden-onset sensorineural hearing loss is often assumed to be due to such an acute event and is an ENT emergency. Treatment consists of bed rest, steroids and in some centres the administration of vasodilators such as carbogen (oxygen and carbon dioxide mixture) or low-molecular-weight dextrans may be employed in an attempt to improve labyrinthine blood flow.

# ACOUSTIC TRAUMA

Most of us have experienced transient acoustic trauma, for example after listening to loud music. The mild hearing loss and tinnitus quickly resolve. However, repeated trauma of this type can cause permanent symptoms. Acute acoustic trauma may also arise from a sudden very loud sound noise, such as an explosion. Although sensorineural deafness due to cochlear damage is the usual consequence, one must also consider the possibility of a conductive deafness due to tympanic membrane rupture or middle ear damage.

Chronic noise-induced hearing loss results from long-term exposure to loud noise. This is most often seen in those who have worked in heavy industry, but may occur in any circumstance where there is repeated exposure to loud noise. Tinnitus is often a

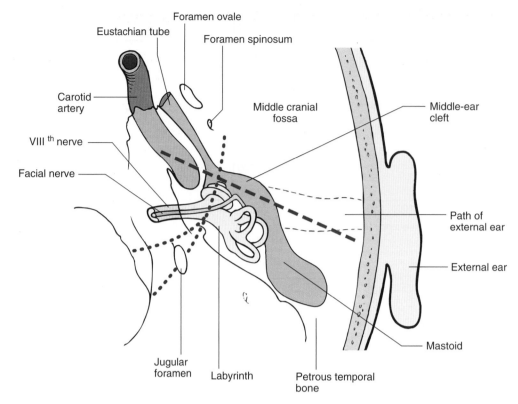

FIGURE 9.28 Temporal bone fractures. ---, pathway of longitudinal fractures; ●●●, pathway of transverse fractures.

prominent feature in this condition and the audiogram has a classical appearance with 'dip' at 4 kHz (Figure 9.27). There are laws governing noise exposure at work and affected individuals can sometimes be eligible for compensation. Prevention is paramount since the treatment is essentially supportive with tinnitus counselling and provision of a hearing aid where necessary.

# TEMPORAL BONE TRAUMA

## Labyrinthine concussion

Hearing loss, tinnitus and vertigo can result from a head injury even if it does not cause a fracture. Pressure waves in the skull base may damage the membranous labyrinth, VIIIth nerve or even the brainstem due to shearing forces as the brain moves relative to the skull. The resulting hearing loss is usually in the high-frequency range and, once more, may occur either with or without tinnitus. It may recover slowly, but unfortunately, can also be permanent.

Vertigo may also occur either due to direct vestibular damage or as a result of otolith displacement. A condition known as 'benign paroxysmal positional vertigo' is thought to result from displacement of otoliths. This is further described later in this chapter.

## Temporal bone fracture

If trauma to the head is severe, a temporal bone fracture may occur. These tend to be either longitudinal (80–90%) or transverse (10–20%) (Figure 9.28).

Transverse fractures usually involve the labyrinth and thus lead to sensorineural hearing loss, often with profound vertigo. This tends to settle in time as central compensation occurs. The hearing loss, however, is permanent. In about 50% of cases there is an associated facial nerve palsy and if this is complete and of immediate onset, early surgical decompression can improve the long-term chances of recovery. However, if the level of consciousness is depressed as a result of a significant brain injury, the palsy may not become apparent until later.

Longitudinal fractures usually spare the labyrinth, although some concussional damage may occur. These fractures involve the external meatus and roof of the middle-ear. Any hearing loss here tends to be conductive, either due to ossicular dislocation, bleeding into the middle-ear cleft or tympanic membrane rupture. Bleeding from the ear and CSF otorrhoea can result especially if the tympanic membrane is disrupted. Facial palsy is uncommon. CSF otorrhoea usually settles spontaneously over a short period of time, during which it is important to be aware of the small risk of meningitis.

A temporal bone fracture must be suspected if there is any bleeding from the ear following head trauma. A high index of suspicion is important since even with high-definition computed tomography (CT) scans, these fractures may be very hard to demonstrate radiologically.

## Round/oval window rupture

Rapid changes in pressure across these labyrinthine membranes, such as may occur with diving, flying, trauma to the ear or sometimes even with coughing or straining, may lead to rupture. In such cases a fluctuating hearing loss with vertigo are the major symptoms. In most, these symptoms will settle with bed rest and vestibular sedatives, but if this does not occur, surgical exploration with identification and closure of the fistula may be required.

# DRUG OTOTOXICITY

Many drugs can damage the inner ear. Some drugs differentially affect the cochlea causing hearing loss and tinnitus, whilst others pick out the vestibular system causing vertigo. Aminoglycosides, such as gentamicin, are well known to be ototoxic, and so are some diuretics, e.g. frusemide, and certain antimalarial drugs, as well as many others. Recognition of risk factors such as poor renal function in patients being treated with an aminoglycoside is most important. Treatment of ototoxicity consists simply in withdrawal of the drug in order to prevent further damage.

Many ear drops contain an aminoglycoside and are used regularly in treating ear infections. There is a small risk of ototoxicity when using these preparations. However, it should be remembered that pus too is ototoxic and also that the infected mucosa of the middle ear is oedematous and as such acts as a physical barrier to diffusion, so reducing the amount of drug that can reach the inner ear. The reality is that short courses of such drops, even in the presence of a tympanic membrane perforation (when infected) are safe and effective. However, prolonged use of such drops in a perforated ear can cause permanent hearing loss and as such should be avoided.

# MÉNIÈRE'S DISEASE

The characteristic triad of symptoms in this condition are *episodic*:

hearing loss – tinnitus – vertigo

Ménière's attacks can occur at any time and last usually from 30 minutes to 24 hours. The vertigo is often disabling and very acute in onset. Nausea and vomiting may also occur and nystagmus is present during attacks. The patient often has to remain in bed until the episode has passed and will often feel a little off balance for the next few days. The hearing loss is sensorineural in type and in the early stages of the disease affects the lower frequencies and returns to normal after the attack. Tinnitus and a feeling of fullness or pressure in the affected ear may precede the attacks.

The disease is usually unilateral initially but can become bilateral. Over the course of the condition, the hearing loss and tinnitus become permanent. These attacks can occur in sporadic bursts or may occur only very occasionally. The unreliability of the attacks and their ability to render patients prostrate often leads to some anxiety and may seriously curtail their daily activities.

Distension of the membranous labyrinth or 'endolymphatic hydrops' is postulated as the underlying cause of this condition. However, the exact aetiology remains unknown. It is thought that attacks occur due to small ruptures in Reissner's membrane leading to mixing of the endo- and perilymph, so causing vertigo which settles as healing occurs. Endolymphatic hydrops can also occur in other conditions of the inner ear such as syphilis, labyrinthitis, head injury and vascular occlusions. However, this tends to be non-progressive, unlike Ménière's disease, which often follows an unremitting course, until the labyrinth is non-functional.

The diagnosis is strongly suggested by the clinical history but it is important to exclude other causes of vertigo such as epilepsy, multiple sclerosis, tumours and vascular disease as well as a labyrinthitis and benign paroxysmal positional vertigo (BPPV). In the acute phase, the treatment of Ménière's disease consists of vestibular sedatives. In the long term, betahistine (a vasodilator), diuretics, avoidance of caffeine and salt, along with reassurance, can help reduce the number of attacks and the patient's ability to cope with attacks. If the disease becomes debilitating, surgery may be considered. This may involve decompressing the endolymphatic sac but sometimes destroying the labyrinth surgically (or chemically) or cutting the VIIIth nerve may be considered.

## CASE STUDY

Vanessa is 38 years old and calls her GP out to her home complaining of dizziness. This is the third time she has been confined to bed with a balance problem and each attack is similar. Initially, she notices a sensation that her right ear is blocked, then this is followed by a rushing noise in her ear and a violent 'sea sickness' sensation. Over the last few months, she has noted that the hearing in her right ear is a little muffled. Examination shows her to be lying flat in bed and reluctant to move her head. She has some nystagmus but the rest of the examination is normal.

1 What is the diagnosis?
2 What is the initial treatment?
3 What is the likely progression of her condition?
4 Does surgery have a role to play?

**Comments**

1 It is highly likely that Vanessa has Ménière's disease. However one should be aware that other conditions can mimic this condition, including acoustic neuromas which may present with Ménière's-like symptoms. She will require full neuro-otological examination and further investigation including an audiogram.

2 Many patients with Ménière's disease find that vestibular sedatives help to reduce the unpleasant dizzy sensation. In order to try to prevent attacks various treatments may be tried including betahistine, diuretics and reducing dietary salt and caffeine.

3 It is likely that her attacks will continue, but with treatment, it is hoped that they will become less frequent and severe. With each attack, it is likely that her hearing will deteriorate a little, with the lower frequencies being most affected. Eventually, her attacks will cease as the disease 'burns out'. The other ear may also become involved at any time.

4 Yes, grommet insertion, saccus surgery, labyrinthectomy and vestibular nerve section are all offered in some centres.

# BENIGN PAROXYSMAL POSITIONAL VERTIGO (BPPV)

This is a condition characterized by episodic vertigo which occurs when the head is moved in certain positions. Classically, it is brought on by turning in bed or looking up at an object, and usually only lasts for minutes but can remain for hours. The episodes of BPPV may occur regularly for weeks or months before slowly settling. It can occur at any age and is probably one of the commonest causes of vertigo. Diagnosis is clinical; the diagnostic bedside test is the 'Hallpike manoeuvre'. Here, the patient sits on a couch facing the examiner. The patient then quickly lies flat and the examiner, supporting the patient's head, turns it through 30° and inclines it downwards. In a positive test, the symptoms are reproduced and nystagmus is observed. The patient sits up, and after a short while, the test is repeated, turning the patient's head towards the opposite side. The nystagmus of BPPV has specific characteristics: it is rotary towards the underlying affected ear, it has a latent period before starting and the nystagmus fatigues (slowly settles) and shows adaptation (lessens with consecutive tests).

BPPV is thought to be caused by dislodged otoliths settling in the posterior semicircular canal, and with certain movements causing irritation of the sensory epithelium, and therefore vertigo. Treatment is with reassurance that the disorder invariably settles spontaneously. A complex series of head manoeuvres which may be performed in the clinic have been described. They attempt to tip the displaced otoliths out of the semicircular canal (Epsley's manoeuvre). In addition, labyrinthine exercises (Cooksey–Cawthorne) can be used to speed up vestibular compensation in this and any other cause of vestibular dysfunction. Vestibular sedatives should be avoided as they will retard the compensation process. Very rarely, surgery on the posterior semicircular canal may be needed.

# VESTIBULAR NEURONITIS

The VIIIth nerve leaves the inner ear via the internal auditory meatus to enter the brain stem at the cerebellopontine angle (CPA). In the brainstem, connections are made with the auditory and vestibular nuclei. Disease processes may affect the VIIIth nerve during its pathway from the cochlea (hence the term 'retrocochlear pathology') leading to hearing loss, vertigo and tinnitus.

Inflammation of the vestibular portion of the VIIIth nerve leads to vertigo with similar symptoms to labyrinthitis. The major cause of this is thought to be a viral infection and the hearing is usually unaffected. Resolution gradually occurs over a period of weeks with slow compensation. Treatment, as with labyrinthitis, consists of vestibular sedatives and rest.

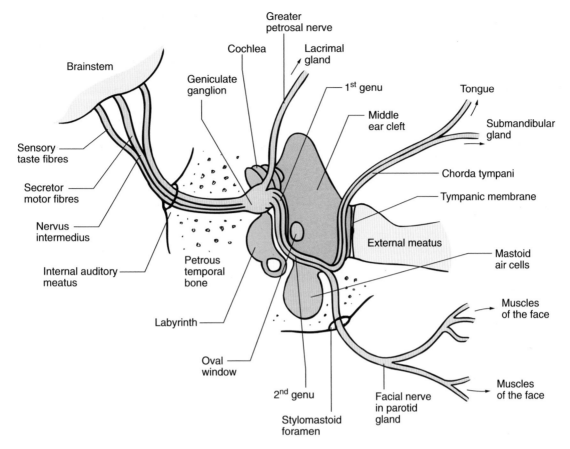

FIGURE 9.29 Schematic diagram of the course of the facial nerve.

# ACOUSTIC NEUROMAS AND CPA TUMOURS

Tumours of the CPA are uncommon but can present with hearing loss, tinnitus and vertigo. Acoustic neuromas, which are actually schwannomas of the vestibular division of VIIIth nerve, are the most common of these lesions, although meningiomas and other intracranial tumours do occur. Slow expansion of the tumour leads to compression of the VIIIth nerve and unilateral otological symptoms. Hence, any patient who presents with unilateral hearing loss or tinnitus, which cannot be explained by another cause, must be investigated further. An MRI scan (Figure 2.7) is the gold standard for diagnosing these tumours which can be very small and difficult to detect when they first start causing symptoms. Treatment is usually by surgical excision, although some tumours can be slow growing and in the elderly, a 'watch and wait' policy may be observed.

# FACIAL NERVE (Figure 9.29)

Neurological diseases may cause or even present with otological symptoms. CNS infections such as meningitis can cause profound deafness, especially in children. Vascular occlusion in the brainstem may lead to vertigo or a hearing loss. Multiple sclerosis can present with vertigo or facial nerve weakness. It is important to consider these disorders especially when there are unilateral otological symptoms and a neurological examination is indicated.

The facial nerve is a motor nerve supplying the muscles of the face. Its nucleus is situated in the pons and the nerve emerges in the cerebellopontine angle. It is associated with the nervus intermedius which carries secretormotor fibres to the salivary glands of the head and neck (except the parotid gland) from the superior salivary nucleus. This nerve also carries the taste fibres from the anterior part of the tongue. The facial nerve enters the internal auditory meatus with the VIIIth nerve and travels through the petrous temporal bone to emerge on the medial surface of the middle ear. Here, the nerve turns posteriorly making its first 'genu' and then turning again, its 'second genu', to travel inferiorly through the mastoid bone and exit the skull at the stylomastoid foramen to supply the facial muscles. The nervus intermedius runs with the facial nerve, giving off the greater petrosal nerve and the chorda tympani (which can be seen travelling on the medial portion of the tympanic membrane), which carries taste fibres from the tongue.

## Facial nerve palsy

Any process that disrupts the nerve fibres of the facial nerve will lead to a partial or total weakness of the facial muscles. This is usually immediately apparent and leads to the patient rapidly seeking medical help because of the obvious cosmetic deformity. It is important to differentiate between an upper motor neurone (UMN) and lower motor palsy (LMN). An UMN palsy is caused by damage to the nerve fibres above the level of the facial nucleus, i.e. the motor cortex or pons. This is distinguished from an LMN palsy by the sparing of movement in the forehead muscles which receive innervation from the contralateral motor cortex as well. An LMN palsy causes total facial weakness (Figure 9.30). A thorough ENT, neck and neurological examination is mandatory for any patient presenting with a facial palsy.

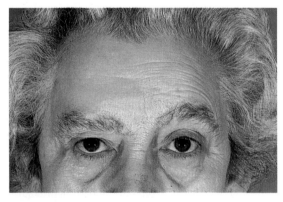

FIGURE 9.30 A lower motor neurone facial nerve palsy. Note the weakness of eyebrow raising and the lack of wrinkles on the affected forehead.

## Bell's palsy

Viral infections that involve the VIIth nerve are possibly one of the commonest causes of facial weakness

### CASE STUDY

Mary is 55 years old and was horrified to find that the left side of her face was 'drooping' when she awoke this morning. She feels well in herself and has no other associated symptoms. Her daughter, who is a nurse, has told her that she has a Bell's palsy.

1 What particular features would you look for in your examination and why?
2 What is the treatment for this condition?

**Comments**

1 Firstly, one must decide if the facial palsy is due to an upper or lower motor neurone lesion. A Bell's palsy will give an LMN pattern, that is to say, the forehead will be involved and hence there is no movement when the patient is asked to raise their eyebrows. One must look for other neurological deficits, especially in the other cranial nerves (including the VIIIth nerve) in order to exclude a systemic neurological condition or an intracranial neoplasm. It is vital that the ear is examined in order to exclude middle-ear disease, such as cholesteatoma. Also, one must look for any vesicles, especially on the ear canal or drum which may suggest a diagnosis of herpetic infection ( Ramsay Hunt syndrome). The parotid must also be examined since the facial nerve traverses this gland and may be damaged by malignant tumours in this area. One must also note the degree of weakness and clearly document this in order that improvement can be monitored. If the patient cannot completely close their eye , they should be referred to the ophthalmic department, due to the danger of corneal ulceration.
2 High-dose oral steroids, if given early, aid recovery. Patients who show no sign of recovery should probably have a scan of the course of the facial nerve in order to exclude any other local cause for such a weakness.

(80%). Bell's palsy probably represents a viral infection of the facial nerve. It presents with a facial palsy, usually of sudden onset, and is often preceded by an upper respiratory tract infection. Increased pressure on the nerve due to swelling in its tight bony canal is thought to be the cause of the dysfunction. If the patient presents within the first 48 hours, treatment with high-dose oral steroids should be considered. The majority of cases resolve completely, but some patients are left with a residual facial weakness. It is a diagnosis of exclusion.

## Trauma

Temporal bone fractures are discussed above and may cause facial weakness. The facial nerve is at risk in surgery on the middle ear, mastoid and parotid gland; therefore, the integrity of the nerve must be checked postoperatively.

## Infection

Infection may damage the facial nerve in the middle ear or more proximally along its course. In some people, the bony fallopian canal that covers the facial nerve in the middle ear may be dehiscent. Acute otitis media in such a case can lead to a facial palsy as the nerve is subject either to pressure or inflammation. Treatment is by antibiotics and decongestants plus sometimes a myringotomy to release the pus. It is important to exclude cholesteatoma as a cause of VIIth nerve palsy which may also present with ear discharge, and may mimic a simple ear infection. 'Malignant' otitis externa (see page 93) also presents with a painful discharging ear and can lead to a facial nerve palsy.

## Ramsay Hunt syndrome

This is caused by the herpes zoster virus. It is characterized by a facial palsy, usually associated with facial pain and the appearance of vesicles on the ear drum, ear canal and pinna. Vertigo and deafness may also occur. Treatment is with acyclovir, an antiviral agent, but this is probably only effective if it is given early in the course of the disease. The facial weakness is usually severe and often does not recover.

## Intracranial causes of facial weakness

These include cerebral ischaemia, multiple sclerosis, cerebellopontine angle lesions and other neurological disorders which may all cause a VIIth nerve palsy.

## Facial nerve tumours

Tumours of the facial nerve itself are rare. The nerve, however, can be involved by a tumour anywhere along its course:

---

> **KEY POINTS**
> ## The Inner Ear
>
> - Presbycusis is the commonset cause of hearing loss in older adults
> - Asymmetric sensorineural hearing loss and tinnitus need further investigation in order to exclude an acoustic neuroma
> - Facial nerve palsy necessitates thorough otoneurological examination

- Parotid gland
    VIIth nerve palsy usually indicates a malignant lesion
- External and middle ear
    Malignant lesions such as sqamous cell carcinoma
- Cerebellopontine angle
    Acoustic neuroma, glomus tumours, etc.
- Petrous Bone
    Cysts, secondary carcinomas

# VERTIGO

Vertigo is an abnormal sensation of movement, and when due to acute vestibular disease, is often rotary in nature. It is important to distinguish true vertigo from unsteadiness, faintness and other types of imbalance from the history. Cardiac and neurological disorders may give symptoms that patients describe as 'dizziness' but are not actually vertiginous in nature. The list below gives many, but not all the causes of vertigo, as well as some conditions that may present as 'dizziness'. The term 'peripheral' is taken to include the ear and labyrinth, whilst central includes the cranial nerves and the brain.

*Peripheral causes*
- Labyrinthitis
- BPPV
- Ménière's disease
- Endolymphatic hydrops from other causes
- Middle-ear diseases
- Post-ear surgery
- Post-trauma
- Vascular insufficiency
- Drugs
- Dead labyrinth from any cause

*Central causes*
- Vestibular neuronitis
- Tumours, e.g. acoustic neuroma
- Multiple sclerosis
- Head injury

- Vascular occlusion
- Drug induced

*Other causes of balance disturbance*
- Cardiac insufficiency
- Cervical spine disease
- Neurological disorders
- Metabolic disorders: diabetes
- Anaemia
- Epilepsy
- Migraine

# TINNITUS

Tinnitus can exist with a hearing loss due to any cause but may occur even with normal hearing. However, it is most often a feature of sensorineural losses. Many people will experience tinnitus at some time in their life, and for most it is a transient and minor problem. However, for some this may become a long-term and troublesome symptom which can trigger depression and even suicide. The noise heard by the patient is usually heard by them alone, termed 'intrinsic', but some tinnitus may be 'extrinsic', and may be heard by an observer, such as a vascular bruit. The list below gives some of the common examples.

Extrinsic causes
- Insects in external ear
- Vascular causes, e.g. arteriovenous malformations/ glomus jugulare tumours
- Palatal myoclonus

Intrinsic causes
*Peripheral*
- Drugs
- Labyrinthitis
- Trauma
- Vascular
- Presbycusis
- Ménière's disease/endolymphatic hydrops
- Noise induced
- Otosclerosis
*Central*
- Idiopathic central tinnitus
- VIIIth nerve tumours
- Temporal lobe epilepsy

## CASE STUDY

Walter is 65 years old, and recently has noted a noise in the right ear. He says it is high pitched, constant and not in time with his pulse. He finds it most distressing and recently has found it difficult to get to sleep as a result of his tinnitus. He says that he has felt a little unsteady on his feet recently, and although he has not noted any hearing loss, an audiogram shows a 40-dB hearing threshold in the right ear with no conductive element to the hearing loss; the left ear is normal.

1   What would be the result of his tuning fork tests?
2   Other than examination of the ears, nose and throat, what else should be examined?
3   Which other investigation should be ordered?

**Comments**
1   Weber test should localize to the better hearing ear in a patient with a unilateral sensorineural hearing loss, in this case the left. Rinne tests will be normal (i.e. positive or AC > BC) in both ears.
2   Full cranial nerve examination including corneal reflexes and fundoscopy are essential, as is testing for cerebellar signs (dysdiadochokinesis, past pointing, etc.). Some form of balance testing such as Romberg's test and/or heal–toe walking should also be performed.
3   The most worrying cause of a unilateral sensorineural hearing loss is an acoustic neuroma. The investigation of choice is an MRI scan of the internal auditory meatus.

# HEARING LOSS

The causes of hearing loss are:

Conductive hearing loss
*External ear*
- Congenital atresia or stenosis
- Meatal obstruction
     foreign bodies
     **wax**
     infection
     keratosis obturans
     neoplasms
*Middle ear*
- Congenital anomaly
     tympanic membrane
     ossicles
     oval/round windows
     cholesteatoma
- **Otitis media**
     acute
     **chronic**
- cholesteatoma

- **Otosclerosis**
- Granulomatous disorders
- Trauma
- Neoplasia

*Sensorineural hearing loss*
*Cochlea*

- Congenital
    dysplasia
    perinatal hypoxia/infection
    syndromic
- **Presbyacusis**
- **Labyrinthitis**/infection
- **Vascular causes**
- Trauma: direct ototoxicity
- **Otosclerosis**
- Ménière's disease/endolymphatic hydrops
- Metabolic disorders
- Haematological disorders

*Retrocochlea*

- Psychogenic
- Meningitis
- Multiple sclerosis
- **Neoplasia, e.g. acoustic neuroma**
- Neurological disorders

# ASSESSMENT OF AUDIOLOGICAL SYMPTOMS

The following flow diagrams give a suggested system which will help the student to come to a differential diagnosis when presented with a patient with a hearing loss or dizziness, or when discussing such cases in an exam situation.

## Diagnosis in hearing loss

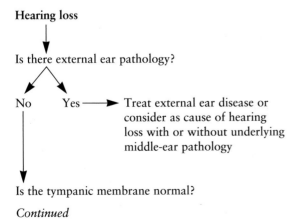

**Hearing loss**

Is there external ear pathology?

No    Yes ⟶ Treat external ear disease or consider as cause of hearing loss with or without underlying middle-ear pathology

Is the tympanic membrane normal?

*Continued*

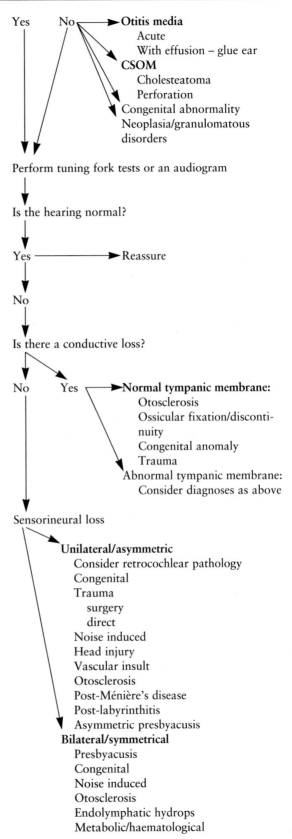

Yes    No ⟶ **Otitis media**
        Acute
        With effusion – glue ear
    **CSOM**
        Cholesteatoma
        Perforation
    Congenital abnormality
    Neoplasia/granulomatous disorders

Perform tuning fork tests or an audiogram

Is the hearing normal?

Yes ⟶ Reassure

No

Is there a conductive loss?

No    Yes ⟶ **Normal tympanic membrane:**
        Otosclerosis
        Ossicular fixation/discontinuity
        Congenital anomaly
        Trauma
    Abnormal tympanic membrane:
        Consider diagnoses as above

Sensorineural loss

    **Unilateral/asymmetric**
        Consider retrocochlear pathology
        Congenital
        Trauma
            surgery
            direct
        Noise induced
        Head injury
        Vascular insult
        Otosclerosis
        Post-Ménière's disease
        Post-labyrinthitis
        Asymmetric presbyacusis
    **Bilateral/symmetrical**
        Presbyacusis
        Congenital
        Noise induced
        Otosclerosis
        Endolymphatic hydrops
        Metabolic/haematological

## Diagnosis in dizziness

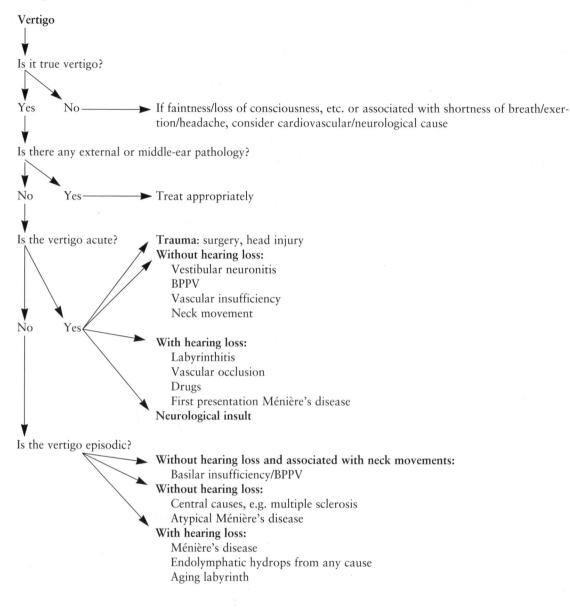

**Vertigo**

Is it true vertigo?

Yes    No——————▶ If faintness/loss of consciousness, etc. or associated with shortness of breath/exertion/headache, consider cardiovascular/neurological cause

Is there any external or middle-ear pathology?

No    Yes——————▶ Treat appropriately

Is the vertigo acute?

No    Yes

**Trauma:** surgery, head injury
**Without hearing loss:**
    Vestibular neuronitis
    BPPV
    Vascular insufficiency
    Neck movement

**With hearing loss:**
    Labyrinthitis
    Vascular occlusion
    Drugs
    First presentation Ménière's disease
**Neurological insult**

Is the vertigo episodic?

**Without hearing loss and associated with neck movements:**
    Basilar insufficiency/BPPV
**Without hearing loss:**
    Central causes, e.g. multiple sclerosis
    Atypical Ménière's disease
**With hearing loss:**
    Ménière's disease
    Endolymphatic hydrops from any cause
    Aging labyrinth

# 10

# The nose and nasopharynx

Structure and function of the nose and
nasopharynx 122

Fractured nose 126

The blocked nose and runny nose 126

Nasal polyposis 132

Growths, tumours and destructive lesions of
the nose 134

Granulomatous and non-granulomatous infection 136

Epistaxis 137

Rhinoplasty and facial plastic surgery 137

The reader must be aware that the sinuses are effectively outpouching of the nasal airway, and that as a result, diseases of the nose may spread to involve the sinuses. Also, sinus disease may present with nasal symptoms. Here, for convenience, the nose and sinuses are described separately, in order that the reader may, piece by piece, build up an overall picture of the system. But, in reality, each is connected to the other anatomically, physiologically and pathologically. Further more, sinonasal tract disease may present with symptoms affecting the ear and oropharynx.

# STRUCTURE AND FUNCTION OF THE NOSE AND NASOPHARYNX

The nose acts as far more than a hole through which we may breathe. In fact, it acts as the air-conditioning unit for the respiratory tract. It also serves to warm and humidify the air that we breathe. Also, it collects moisture from the expired air and so prevents excessive water loss from the respiratory tract. Stiff hairs which grow at the nasal vestibule filter large, potentially harmful particles from the air. Smaller particles are deposited on the lining of the nose and here enzymatic destruction of bacteria and viruses occurs. The epithelial lining of the nose is ciliated and the resulting mucociliary pathway clears nasal debris to the mouth, also helping to lubricate the oropharynx prior to it being swallowed. The nasal cavity and sinuses together give a resonant quality to the voice and the olfactory receptors are sited here also. The nose also houses the olfactory epithelium high up in the olfactory cleft. It is important to recognize that olfaction gives 85% of what we call 'taste', since patients will often say they have a 'poor sense of taste' rather than a 'poor sense of smell'.

## The external nose

The skeleton of the nose is made of bone and cartilage, the upper one-third consists of the nasal bones which are attached to the forehead (frontal bone) and cheeks (maxilla). The lower two-thirds of the nasal skeleton is cartilaginous, the two main components of which are known as the upper and lower lateral cartilages (Figure 10.1). The lower laterals are also known as the alar cartilages. This skeleton is covered with skin which is thin over the nasal bridge and thicker with more sebaceous glands over the nasal tip. Hypertrophy of these glands causes a rhinophyma (Figure 10.2).

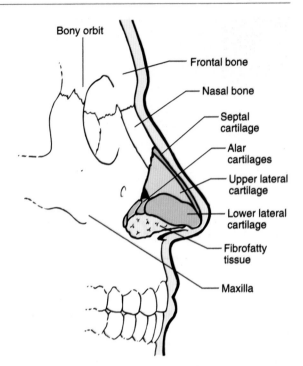

FIGURE 10.1 The skeleton of the external nose.

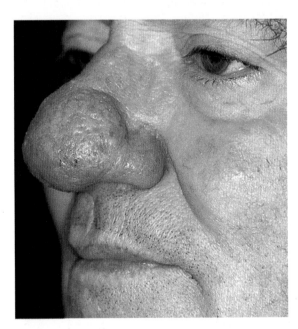

FIGURE 10.2 Rhinophyma.

## The nasal vestibule and nasal valve

The vestibule of the nose is the entrance to the nasal cavity. It is enclosed by the alar cartilages. The skin in this region bears stiff hairs called the vibrissae. The

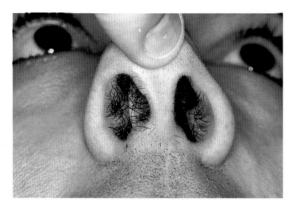

FIGURE 10.3 Columella dislocation – deviation of the free, anterior edge of the nasal septum.

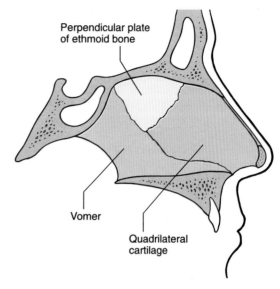

FIGURE 10.4 Anatomy of the nasal septum.

mucous membranes of the nasal cavity lie just behind this hair-bearing skin; the change from one to the other is known as the mucocutaneous junction. Both benign papillomas, basal cell carcinomas as well as malignant squamous cell carcinomas can develop within the nasal vestibule. The midline strip of skin which connects the upper lip to the nasal tip is called the columella. Normally the 'free' caudal edge of the cartilaginous septum lies under the columella. However, occasionally the septum is deviated away from the midline and this free edge can be seen projecting into one vestibule. This is known as a columella dislocation (Figure 10.3)

The narrowest part of the nasal cavity is the nasal valve. This is an area just behind the vestibule, level with the upper border of the alar cartilage. In some patients, especially in later life when the tissues become more lax, the alar cartilage at the level of the nasal valve becomes sucked in during inspiration and causes nasal obstruction. This is known as alar collapse, and when severe, patients may benefit from some form of nasal splinting device in order to prevent this collapse.

## The nasal septum

This is the midline division between each nasal cavity. It is made of thin, flat bony sheets posteriorly and cartilage anteriorly (Figure 10.4). The lower end of the septum sits in a groove in the crest of the maxilla. The maxillary bone makes up the majority of the floor of the nasal cavity. The septum is often slightly deviated into one or other nasal cavities. However if this is a pronounced feature it can cause nasal obstruction (Figure 10.5). The covering of the septum is called mucoperichondrium (when it overlies cartilage) and mucoperiostium (when it overlies the bony component

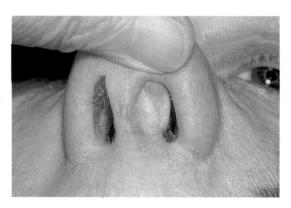

FIGURE 10.5 A gross deviation of the anterior nasal septum, causing left-sided nasal obstruction. Published with the kind permission of Mr G. Bates FRCS.

of the septum). The septum has a rich blood supply, especially anteriorly where four arteries anastomose. This is known as Little's area, and is the most common site for nose bleeds (Figure 10.6).

## The lateral nasal wall

Lateral to the nasal cavity lie the orbit, the maxillary and ethmoid sinuses. These are separated from the nasal cavity by bony sheets which in places are paper thin. Three cigar-shaped ridges or swellings are attached to the lateral nasal wall. These are the superior, middle and inferior turbinates. Each is made of a bone which is covered in vascular mucoperiostium

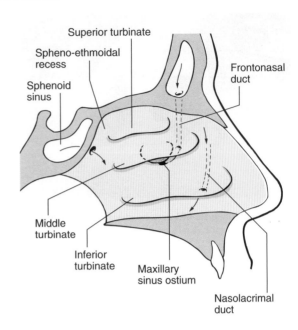

FIGURE 10.6 Blood supply of Little's area and nasal septum.

FIGURE 10.7 Drainage of the nasolacrimal duct and sinuses.

and ciliated columnar epithelium. The space under each turbinate is called a meatus (the inferior meatus lies under the inferior turbinate, etc.). The naso-lacrimal duct and sinuses drain into these spaces (Figure 10.7). The middle meatus is the most important clinically since it is most often affected by disease and the majority of the sinuses drain into it.

The vascular inferior turbinate contains the second most erectile tissue in the body. As a result, it has the ability to swell and shrink under autonomic nervous system control. The function of the inferior turbinates is to control the passage of air through the nose via the nasal cycle. Here the inferior turbinate on one side is enlarged, and as a result the air flow through that nostril is restricted. This reduces the drying effect of air flow and allows for rejuvenation of the nasal lining and ciliary function. After approximately 4 hours, the turbinate on the other side swells and on the previously rested side the turbinate shrinks. This nasal cycle is a normal physiological mechanism which is present to some extent in all of us, but noticed only by some.

## The postnasal space or nasopharynx

The nasal cavities end at the posterior end of the septum as two oval spaces, sometimes referred to as the choanae. Behind this, the nasal cavities are continuous with another space called the nasopharynx or post-nasal space (PNS). Rarely, a congenital anomaly

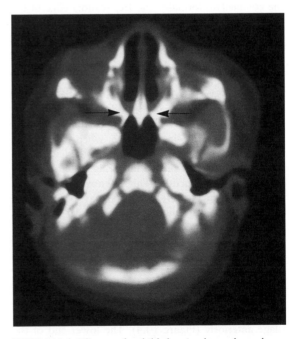

FIGURE 10.8 A CT scan of a child showing bony choanal atresia bilaterally. Published with the kind permission of Mr A.P. Freeland FRCS.

occurs known as choanal atresia. Here a membrane lies across one or both choanae. If bilateral, this condition will be rapidly fatal soon after birth, since

## KEY POINTS
### The Nose and Sinuses

- The nose warms and humidifies the air that we breathe
- The sinuses are outpouchings of the nose. Therefore, diseases which affect one often have secondary effects on the other
- Most of the sinuses drain into the middle meatus
- The eustachian tubes open into the postnasal space. When these are affected by disease, a middle-ear effusion may occur and the patient will usually notice a deterioration in their hearing

neonates are obligate nose breathers and will die unless the attending medical staff insert an oral airway in order to bypass this obstruction (Figure 10.8).

The PNS is clinically relevant since the eustachian tubes open into it on each side. An infected or enlarged adenoid and tumours of the PNS can interfere with eustachian tube function. Similarly, a constant stream of infected nasal secretions washing over the eustachian cushions as they are cleared from the nose can induce secondary inflammation in the eustachian tube. Eustachian tube dysfunction can cause a middle-ear effusion and hearing loss. This may be the sole presenting feature of a nasopharyngeal carcinoma. Therefore, if unilateral, this condition must be investigated further. The nasopharynx is continuous inferiorly with the oropharynx. The dividing line between the two is taken as the level of the soft palate.

## OVERVIEW
### Conditions Affecting the Nose

**Congenital**
- Nasal Agenesis
- Dysmorphic Nose
- **Choanal Atresia**
- Tumours
      Meningocoele, encephalocoele, glioma, dermoid

**Acquired**
*The External Nose*
- **Nasal bone fracture**
- **Skin tumours**
      **Papilloma, basal cell carcinoma, squamous cell carcinoma**
- Rhinophyma

- Vestibular stenosis
- **Vestibulitis**

*The Nasal Cavity*

**Foreign body/rhinolith**

**Rhinitis**
- **Infective**
      Viral, bacterial, fungal
- **Seasonal allergic**
- **Perennial allergic**
- **Vasomotor**
- Atrophic
- **Medicamentosa**

**Polyposis**
- **Simple**
- **Aspirin sensitivity, asthma, nasal polyps triad**
- **Cystic fibrosis**

**Neoplastic**
*Benign*
- **Squamous papilloma**
- **Inverted papilloma**
- Angioma
- Fibroma
- Osteoma

*Malignant*
- **Squamous carcinoma**
- **Adenocarcinoma**
- T-cell lymphoma
- Malignant melanoma
- Olfactory neuroblastoma
- Oncocytoma

**Granulomatous**
- Tuberculosis
- Syphilis
- Scleroma
- **Sarcoidosis**
- **Wegener's granulomatosis**

*The Nasopharynx or Postnasal Space*

**Neoplasia**
- **Carcinoma**
- **Angiofibroma**
- Chordoma
- Craniopharyngioma
- Plasmacytoma
- Rhabdomyosarcoma

## FRACTURED NOSE (Figure 10.9)

Trauma to the external nose is common and 'fractured nose' or 'query fractured nose' are common reasons for referral to the ENT department. Prior to referral, however, one must consider a number of important factors, i.e.

■ Could the patient have suffered a cervical spine injury?
■ Has the patient suffered a significant head injury, the management of which must take priority over the nasal injury?
■ Has there been any other facial injury or fracture which also needs treatment?

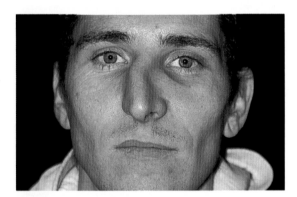

FIGURE 10.9 Gross deviation of the nasal skeleton following nasal fracture.

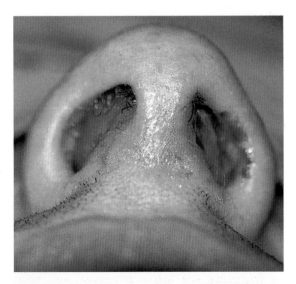

FIGURE 10.10 Septal haematoma following a fractured nose.

■ Is there any chance that the patient may pursue legal action as a result of their injury? if so, take an X-ray of the nasal bones.
■ Is there a septal haematoma? (complete nasal obstruction and characteristic appearances; Figure 10.10).

Once these factors have been determined, one may follow the protocol suggested for the management of a suspected broken nose shown in Figure 10.11.

## THE BLOCKED NOSE AND RUNNY NOSE

A variety of different conditions may cause a sensation of nasal obstruction with or without rhinorrhoea. Broadly speaking, these symptoms may be due to a structural/anatomical abnormality or a mass within the nose, or be due to swelling of the nasal lining due to some inflammatory stimulus. Not infrequently, a combination of pre-existing structural abnormality and a mild inflammatory reaction leads to the development of symptoms. Once again, a carefully taken history will usually guide one towards the diagnosis and a thorough examination will reveal any physical abnormality. Tests of nasal function may be useful in documenting the degree of disability due to nasal pathology. Also, allergy and ciliary-function testing may help to confirm the cause of a suspected lining problem. The details of these tests are covered in Chapter 2.

Features of nasal symptoms which may suggest their cause are as follows:

■ Structural abnormality
    Long history
    Constant
    Usually unilateral or worse on one side
    Previous nasal trauma
    Snoring/sleep apnoea
■ Lining inflammation
    Sneezing
    Nasal itch
    Hayfever
    Asthma
    Bilateral
    Rhinorrhoea
    Postnasal drip
    Pet allergy
    Dust allergy
    Provoking factors

The causes of the blocked/runny nose are discussed in more detail below. This is not an exhaustive account but aims to deal with the most frequently encountered or important causes.

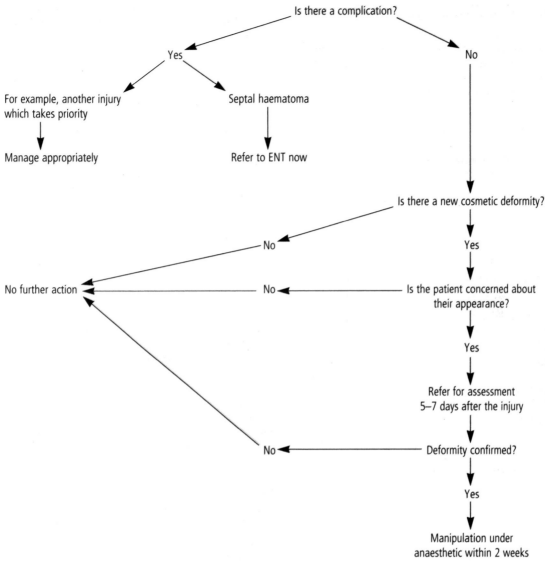

FIGURE 10.11 Management of a suspected broken nose.

## Structural/physical causes of nasal obstruction

### Nasal foreign body

This commonly occurs in young children and a huge variety of objects are known to have been inserted. Most foreign bodies in the nasal cavity elicit a profuse inflammatory response and foul nasal discharge frequently develops within a matter of days; organic materials particularly behave in this way. Frequently the object is inserted without the parents' knowledge, and may remain asymptomatic until a discharge develops. For this reason, a unilateral discharge, particularly in a child, must be assumed to be due to a foreign body, and examination of the nose, under general anaesthesia if necessary, is indicated. A secondary inflammation of the nasal vestibular skin (vestibulitis) may develop in response to the constant discharge (Figure 10.12).

Small (usually non-organic) foreign objects may lie unnoticed in the nose for years. In this case, nasal secretions may solidify around the object and a nasal concretion, or rhinolith, may develop. These can reach an impressive size before presenting with nasal obstruction and/or epistaxis.

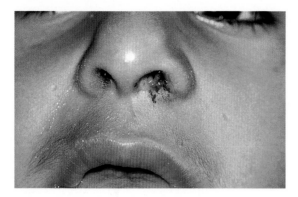

FIGURE 10.12 Unilateral blood-stained nasal discharge in a child is highly suggestive of a nasal foreign body.

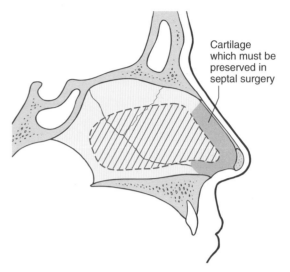

Cartilage which must be preserved in septal surgery

FIGURE 10.13 Area of septum excised in submucus resection (SMR).

## CASE STUDY

Tom is 3 years old, and for the last week has had a runny nose, but only from the left side. Over the last couple of days, his mother has complained that he 'smells awful' and the discharge from the nose is now a little blood-stained.

1   What is the diagnosis?
2   How and when should he be treated?

**Comments**

1   Tom has all the features of a foreign body in his nose.
2   The object must be removed, under general anaesthesia if necessary. There is a theoretical risk of inhalation of the object into the lower respiratory tract. Therefore the object should be removed as soon as this can be arranged.

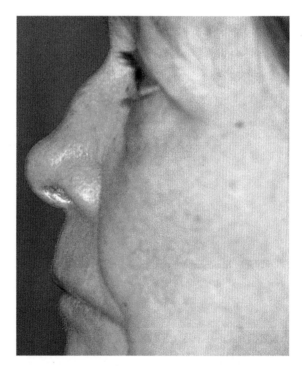

FIGURE 10.14 Saddling of the nasal dorsum leading to supratip depression following excessive cartilage removal during septal surgery some years previously.

## The septum

### Septal deviation

This may result from trauma, either during descent down the birth canal, or from direct nasal trauma in later life. It is also believed that differential rates of growth between the nasal septum and the rest of the mid-face, may lead to a buckling of the septum in some cases. Deviation of the septum, either at its caudal end (columella dislocation) or further back in the nasal cavity can lead to symptomatic nasal obstruction.

### Septal surgery

This aims to correct this deflection of the septum by either removing the deviated cartilage/bone (submucus resection or SMR) or by mobilizing and repositioning the deviated cartilaginous septum (septoplasty). In reality, it is often necessary to excise some, and reposition other parts of the septum in the same operation. Thus, the distinction between these two procedures is more imagined than real. It is important to realize, however, that the surgeon should not excise the anterior or dorsal septum (Figure 10.13) since this provides support for the nose and ugly cosmetic deformities may result (Figure 10.14).

### Septal perforation

This may result from a number of causes:

- Trauma
    Surgical
    Nose picking
- Avascular necrosis
    Secondary to cocaine abuse
    Secondary to septal haematoma or abscess
    Sickle cell disease
- Granulomatous inflammation
    Wegener's granulomatosis
    Syphilis
    Tuberculosis
    Sarcoidosis
- Tumours of the nasal cavity
    T-cell lymphoma = lethal midline granuloma

The resulting distortion of air-flow through the nose can lead to a sense of nasal obstruction. Other symptoms include whistling, crusting and epistaxis.

### Septal haematoma

This occurs in two circumstances: either after septal surgery or as a complication of blunt nasal trauma. Blood accumulates between the cartilage and mucoperichondrium of the septum. As a result, the septum swells dramatically and fills the nasal cavity; total nasal obstruction results. This is an important condition to recognize since, if not treated immediately, avascular necrosis of the cartilaginous septum will result, with collapse of the nose (see Figure 10.14). Infection of such a haematoma will lead to a septal abscess, a condition which even more readily destroys cartilage.

### Choanal atresia

This has been mentioned earlier in this chapter (pages 124–125). However, if this condition affects only one side, it may go unrecognized for many years and rarely may present in adulthood with unilateral nasal obstruction.

## Rhinitis

Rhinitis may be defined as an inflammation of the nasal lining. Most causes of rhinitis lead to broadly similar symptoms, namely nasal congestion, rhinorrhoea, postnasal drip, sneezing and nasal irritation. The history and allergy tests usually give the best indication of the cause of the rhinitis.

## Simple acute infective rhinitis

This is well known to all of us as the nasal effects of the common cold. It is usually viral in origin, spread by droplet transmission and is mild and self-limiting. Occasionally, the secondary effects of a cold can persist after the instigating infection has passed. For example, a middle-ear effusion (secretory otitis media) or long-running sinusitis which usually develops as a result of secondary bacterial infection. Other specific nasal infections such as syphilis, tuberculosis and scleroma are covered below.

## Allergic rhinitis

This is probably the second most common type of rhinitis. Here the nasal lining becomes sensitive to particular tiny particles known as allergens. When these allergens are absorbed into the nasal mucous membrane they cause a hypersensitivity reaction (Type 1, IgE-mediated response (see Figure 10.15)); as a result,

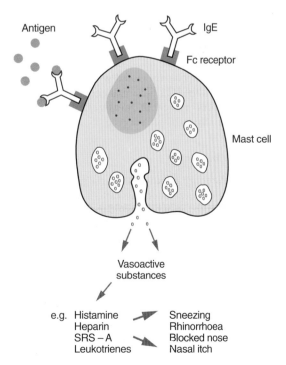

FIGURE 10.15 Type 1 hypersensitivity reaction (mast cell degranulation).

TABLE 10.1 Common allergens associated with allergic rhinitis

| ROUTE | COMMON ALLERGENS | TYPE OF ALLERGIC RHINITIS |
|---|---|---|
| Inhaled | Pollen | Seasonal |
| | House dust | |
| | Dust mite | |
| | Animal dander | |
| | Feathers | Perennial |
| Ingested | Wheat | |
| | Eggs | |
| | Milk | |
| | Nuts | |

a range of vasoactive substances, such as histamine, are released, and together they cause the typical local effects of nasal allergy – vascular congestion, oedema, rhinorrhoea and irritation.

Some patients are allergic to certain allergens which are only present in a particular season, e.g. grass pollens or fungal spores which are released during summer or autumn. As a result, the patient will only suffer from rhinitis at this particular time of year; this is *seasonal rhinitis*, commonly known as hayfever. Here the patient also frequently complains of watery itchy eyes.

In perennial rhinitis, the same response occurs but to different allergens which are prominent all year round, for example house dust and house dust mite. Examination of the nose in these patients will often reveal a damp, pale nasal lining with swollen oedematous turbinates. In long-standing nasal allergy, the turbinates often become hypertrophied and permanently enlarged and lose much of their erectile ability.

Common allergens associated with allergic rhinitis are listed in Table 10.1. The management of allergic rhinitis involves avoidance measures, drug therapy and occasionally turbinate surgery.

### Allergen avoidance

These measures are effective when the patient is allergic to a single allergen and this can be identified. The common allergens in which avoidance is possible are house dust, house dust mite and animal hair allergy. Here simple measures such as regularly vacuuming the bedding, washing the sheets and avoiding close contact with pets are helpful if the patient can be persuaded to comply with them.

### Drug therapy

This aims to modify or damp down the allergic response. The commonly used drugs are outlined below. Those who wish to know more should refer to Chapter 14 on pharmacology and ENT.

■ *Steroid preparations:* These are most often employed, either as topical sprays or drops, or in severe cases as oral or depot injections. Steroids often need to be taken on a long-term basis, since they control rather than cure patients' symptoms.
■ *Antihistamines:* These are now available both as non-sedating oral preparations as well as topical nasal sprays.
■ *Sodium cromoglycate nasal spray:* This is effective in stabilizing mast cells, but has to be used 4–6 times a day. It is useful in children and those patients who are unhappy about taking steroids, despite explanation that topical steroids have little or no side effects, even when used long term.

## Vasomotor rhinitis

This is a condition which has, in the past, been used as a diagnosis of exclusion. The symptoms are similar to allergic rhinitis, and indeed swabs of the nose show eosinophilia as in allergic rhinitis. However, the patient frequently fails to test positive for the common allergens. Some take this to mean that we have simply failed to identify the allergen responsible, while others believe that this represents a truly separate condition. There does seem to be a relatively small group of patients who give a convincing history of nasal symptoms in response to positional and climatic factors, such as a sudden change in temperature. Similarly, some patients seem to have symptoms triggered by alcohol or emotional changes.

Thankfully, we do not need to concern ourselves further since the treatment for this condition is similar to that for true allergic rhinitis, i.e. avoidance of any known precipitating factors and nasal steroid preparations. In patients whose primary complaint is of watery rhinorrhoea, the anticholinergic ipratropium bromide, delivered as a nasal spray, is often effective. In resistant cases with turbinate hypertrophy (see below), surgery may indicated.

## Rhinitis medicamentosa

This is an acquired sensitivity of the nasal lining in response to the prolonged use of topical nasal decongestant substances. The root of the problem lies in the fact that, once the effect of a nasal decongestant has worn off, there is a rebound vasodilatation. This leads to further nasal congestion, the patient feels the need for relief and so uses the decongestant again. The whole process rapidly becomes self-perpetuating and results in turbinate hypertrophy with chronic, unresponsive nasal obstruction. Many over-the-counter preparations contain nasal decongestants and these must be enquired about directly when taking the history, since patients will rarely offer this information spontaneously.

Prevention by education of patients is important. Treatment involves cessation of the decongestants, with instigation of topical nasal steroids, and where turbinate hypertrophy is a major feature, turbinate resection may be required.

## Atrophic rhinitis

This condition was much more frequent in the past and is seen more often in developing countries. It would seem therefore that socio-economic factors have some role to play in the development of this condition.

Nowadays, in the West, atrophic rhinitis is associated with an abnormal patency of the nostril, usually as a result of nasal surgery, particularly turbinate resection. The nasal lining looses its cilia and atrophies. Thick secretions are formed which quickly dry and lead to large crusts which have a characteristic unpleasant odour. Bleeding is frequent. Nasal toilet is required regularly, and the patient is encouraged to use steam inhalations and glucose in glycerin nose drops in an attempt to soften the crusts. The most effective treatment is surgically to close off the nostril. However, this is often poorly tolerated by the patient. With the cessation of air flow, the nasal lining returns to normal, but when the airway is re-opened, the problem returns.

## Other types of rhinitis

These have been described in response to a wide variety of factors. Some of these include:

### Rhinitis of pregnancy

This occurs in response to the hormonal changes associated with childbearing. The condition resolves after parturition.

### Senile rhinitis or dew drop nose

This describes the watery anterior rhinorrhoea which occurs particularly in old men.

### Honeymoon rhinitis

This refers to nasal symptoms which occur as a result of sexual excitation.

### Rhinitis sicca

This occurs as a result of exposure to extremely hot dry conditions, such as in foundry workers or in the desert.

## Turbinate surgery

This is performed in cases of permanent turbinate hypertrophy. Turbinates may either be excised (totally or partially), or scarring of the vascular turbinate tissue can be induced, with resulting shrinkage. Many different scarring techniques are employed, which largely depends on the surgeon's personal preference. Hot wire, cryotherapy and laser cautery are all used to scar the surface of the turbinate. Submucus diathermy (SMD) and filleting of the turbinate bone are used in order to cause subepithelial scarring (Figure 10.16). The immediate risk is of bleeding. This can be impressive and potentially life-threatening at times. Later atrophic rhinitis can develop, usually after radical turbinate excision. Even minor intervention/surgery to the nose can lead to nasal adhesions. Here the inferior turbinate becomes stuck to the nasal septum (Figure 10.17). This may cause nasal obstruction if severe, but often such adhesions are asymptomatic. Treatment is by division of the adhesions.

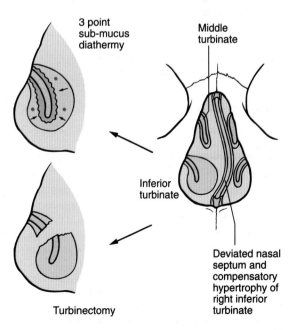

FIGURE 10.16 Turbinate surgery.

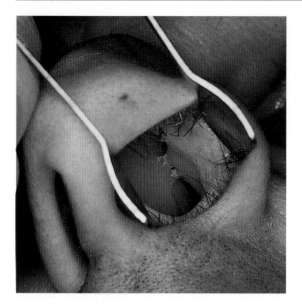

FIGURE 10.17 Nasal adhesions.

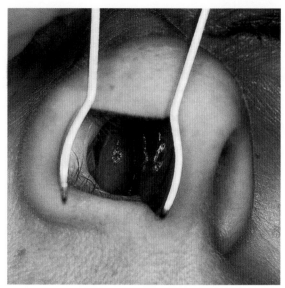

FIGURE 10.18 Nasal polyp - note the translucent grey appearance. Polyps are mobile on probing; the turbinates are not.

---

### KEY POINTS
#### Rhinitis

- The most common types of rhinitis are: infective (a cold); and allergic. Allergic rhinitis may be either seasonal or perennial
- Most types of rhinitis will give similar symptoms, i.e. nasal blockage, rhinorrhoea and sneezing
- In allergic rhinitis the main treatment options are allergen avoidance and steroids which may be administered systemically or topically
- Long-standing rhinitis can cause the turbinates to hypertrophy. In this case, turbinate surgery may be required

---

# NASAL POLYPOSIS

A nasal polyp is simply a descriptive term for a pedunculated swelling arising in the nose or paranasal sinuses. Polyps may develop in both benign and malignant conditions. In this section, we shall deal with those simple inflammatory polyps which are most common. Other types of polyps which may herald malignant disease will be discussed later in this chapter. Simple inflammatory polyps are usually bilateral and therefore a unilateral polyp must be biopsied in order to exclude malignancy. Prolapse of the meninges (meningocoele) or brain tissue (encephalocoele) can

occur through the roof of the nasal cavity and may mimic such a polyp. Obviously, this must be excluded prior to biopsy.

## Features of nasal polyposis

As with most benign nasal pathology, the symptoms include nasal obstruction, anosmia and anterior rhinorrhoea, but the diagnosis is usually easy to make on examination of the nose. Simple polyps are usually seen bilaterally and tend to occupy the middle meatus because they arise within the ethmoid sinuses which drain into this region of the nose. They are grey/white and often appear slightly translucent (Figure 10.18). They are soft and mobile on gentle probing, unlike the middle or inferior turbinates which are frequently misdiagnosed as polyps by the inexperienced (Figure 10.19). Large polyps may expand the nose and when they prolapse through the nostril often become fleshy and ulcerated. Polyps which bleed, look suspicious or are unilateral must be biopsied.

## Associated disorders

The exact cause of nasal polyps remains uncertain. However, certain associations between nasal polyps and other diseases have been noted. The triad of *aspirin–sensitivity–asthma* and nasal polyps is well recognized and tends to be associated with fulminant

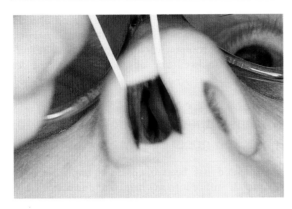

FIGURE 10.19 Note the anterior end of the middle turbinate which can be seen projecting from the side wall of the nasal cavity. This is often confused with a nasal polyp by the less experienced.

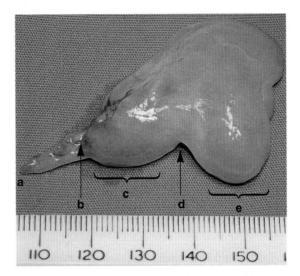

FIGURE 10.20 (a) The point of attachment to the mucosa of the maxillary sinus; (b) a narrowing corresponding to the ostium of the maxillary sinus; (c) portion of the polyp lying within the middle meatus; (d) a narrowing representing the posterior choana; (e) portion of the polyp which occupies the nasopharynx.

aggressive disease. Also childhood polyposis must raise the question of unrecognized *cystic fibrosis*. Nasal allergy was thought for many years to be responsible for the development of polyps. However, recently, it has been shown that the prevalence of nasal allergy is no higher in polyp patients than in the healthy population. Infection has been suspected by some for many years, but only recently has an association been made between *Mycoplasmal infection* and nasal polyposis.

## Treatment

### Medical treatments

Medical therapy for nasal polyposis includes antihistamines and nasal decongestants (used sparingly). However, the mainstay of medical therapy is steroids. These may be applied as a topical spray or more effectively as nasal drops instilled in the head-down position. In severe cases, a 'medical polypectomy' is required. This will include combination topical agents as well as a short course of oral steroids, and is often very effective.

Once polyps have been controlled, either by medical or surgical means, maintenance therapy with long-term inhaled steroids is recommended.

### Surgical treatments

The surgical treatments for nasal polyps consist in simple intranasal polypectomy or in severe/recurrent cases it may be necessary to open the ethmoid sinuses in order to allow complete removal of the polyps. This also has the effect of allowing the nasal steroids to

enter this area easily after surgery. Such an ethmoidectomy may be performed through the nose or via an external approach (see Figure 11.13, p. 146).

## Antro-choanal polyp

Antro-choanal polyp is the name given to a particular type of benign solitary polyp which originates from the mucosa of the maxillary antrum. It is uncommon but occurs most frequently in young men. As it enlarges, the polyp extends through the maxillary sinus ostium and into the nasal cavity. From here, it

### KEY POINTS
#### Nasal Polyps

- Simple inflammatory polyps tend to be bilateral; a unilateral nasal polyp must be biopsied
- An ulcerated or bleeding nasal polyp must be biopsied
- Polyps move on gentle probing; the turbinates do not
- Simple polyps should be treated with steroids, either orally or topically
- Polyps resistant to medical treatment may need to be surgically removed, but they tend to recur. The remission period can be extended by the use of long-term topical nasal steroids

## CASE STUDY

Sylvia, a 55-year-old receptionist, complains of a nasal quality to her voice, as well as a blocked and runny nose. She has never had a very good nasal airway. However, recently her symptoms have become much more pronounced. She now has lost her sense of taste and smell, and after colds she suffers with mid-facial aches and pains for some weeks. She also complains of postnasal drip. She has recently been diagnosed as having asthma and has been started on oral steroid inhalers. Examination confirms the paucity of her nasal airway and polyp-like swellings within the nose on both sides.

1  What are the features of nasal polyps on examination?
2  What should be the first line of treatment in this lady?
3  What specific enquiry should be made as part of the drug history?
4  When should she be referred for surgery?

**Comments**

1  Simple inflammatory nasal polyps are nearly always bilateral and tend to arise from the middle meatus. They are usually pale grey and translucent on examination. However, if they are so large as to prolapse out of the nose, the exposed area can undergo metaplasia and become thickened and red. Polyps are insensate, soft and mobile on probing; the turbinates are not.
2  Since there is no history of previous polyp formation, and the appearances are highly suggestive of a simple inflammatory polyps, it would be reasonable to try a course of topical steroids, either as a spray or drop formulation, administered in the head-down position. In some severe cases, a short course of oral steroids is helpful in a achieving maximal response quickly.
3  Is there any history of an adverse reaction to aspirin? Remember the ASA triad.
4  Surgery should be considered if simple polyps fail to respond to properly applied topical steroids. Any unilateral polyp or those which have atypical appearances or bleed, must be biopsied in order to exclude neoplasia.

expiration. If extremely large, it can extend into the mouth. Treatment is via simple avulsion and removal of the antral component through the nose (Figure 10.20). A Caldwell–Luc approach is reserved for recurrent cases.

## Postnasal space conditions leading to a blocked nose

The adenoid has been discussed in more detail in Chapter 3. Suffice it to say here, that an enlarged adenoid can severely impinge upon the nasal airway. An affected child will suffer with rhinorrhoea, mouth breathing, may struggle when eating due to their poor nasal airway and may snore or suffer with sleep apnoea.

PNS tumours of any kind may interfere with the nasal airway and so may present as a blocked nose as part of their symptomatology. These lesions are discussed in more detail below.

# GROWTHS, TUMOURS AND DESTRUCTIVE LESIONS OF THE NOSE

Few areas of the body have such a diversity of possible pathologies, all of which present with broadly similar features. It is far beyond the scope of this book to describe fully each of these conditions. We shall, however, try to give a structured outline of the important diseases.

The presenting features of sinonasal tumours are as follows:

■ Common
  Nasal obstruction, usually unilateral
  Unilateral blood-stained nasal discharge
  Epistaxis
  A lump in the nose
■ Less common
  Facial swelling
  Proptosis
  Neck lump
  Facial pain/paraesthesia

## Benign neoplasms

### Simple papillomas (or viral warts)

These tend to occur in the nasal vestibule and may mimic a squamous cell carcinoma. They should be excised and sent for histological examination.

progresses posteriorly towards the nasopharynx. Once in the region of the posterior choana, it can exert a ball-valve effect, with unilateral nasal obstruction on

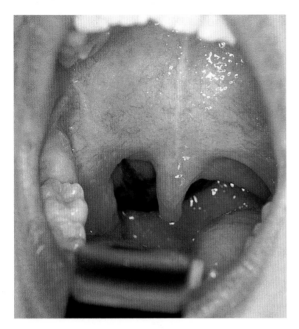

FIGURE 10.21 An angiofibroma presenting as a swelling hanging down from the postnasal space and projecting into the mouth. Do not biopsy this vascular tumour.

## Inverted papilloma

This is the common name for *transitional cell papilloma*. It derives its name from the histological appearance of its surface which appears infolded. The tumour is frequently multicentric and may appear similar to a simple inflammatory nasal polyp. Recurrence is common and malignant change occurs in some cases. Therefore, the tumour should be removed *in toto*.

## Juvenile angiofibroma

This is a tumour of adolescent boys, arising in the nasopharynx. This is an extremely vascular neoplasm which may present with profuse epistaxis on a background of unilateral nasal obstruction. A computed tomography scan is vital to assess any intracranial extension. The tumour must not be biopsied prior to complete surgical excision and this should only be attempted by the most experienced and fearless head and neck surgeons. Pre-operative embolization of the feeder blood vessels is favoured by many in order to reduce the operative haemorrhage (Figure 10.21) and in some centres, primary radiotherapy is advocated.

## Malignant neoplasms

### Squamous cell carcinoma

This is the commonest malignant tumour of the nose and sinuses, and like other malignant tumours of the nasal cavity, tends to arise from the lateral nasal wall. It was common in the nickel industry before industrial exposure to this carcinogen was regulated. The tumour may invade the sinuses, orbit, brain, cheek and palate. It tends to be spread by the lymph system. Combined surgical excision and radiotherapy is the treatment of choice, but results are poor with only 30% of patients surviving beyond five years.

### Adenocarcinoma

Adenocarcinoma also occurs in the nose and a causative link to industrial exposure to hardwood dust has been proven.

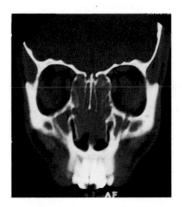

(a)

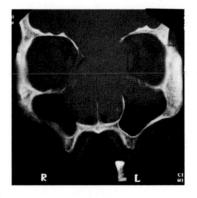

(b)

FIGURE 10.22 (a) CT scan showing the typical appearances of benign nasal polyps. Note the opacifications of the ethmoids and the preservation of the bone of the septum and middle turbinates. Compare this to (b): a CT scan showing a malignant nasal tumour. Note the widespread bone destruction and spread beyond the nasal cavity.

## CASE STUDY

Chin is a 43-year-old researcher who rather reluctantly presents complaining of a lump in his left neck. He says it has been present for 'a long time' and finds it difficult to be any more precise. Although he does not admit to any other symptoms, his wife says that he has started snoring recently and she thinks he is going deaf. Examination of his neck reveals a firm 2 cm $\times$ 2 cm mass just below the angle of the left mandible.

1   What is the most likely diagnosis?
2   Give three other potential causes for such a lump.
3   Malignancies of which sites commonly give rise to cervical lymph node metastases?

**Comments**

1   Nasopharyngeal carcinoma. This is more common amongst the Chinese population. It often causes few symptoms until it metastasizes. However, glue ear due to eustachian tube involvement, and nasal obstruction or epistaxis occur with more advanced disease.
2   Possibilities include:
   ■ Metastatic carcinoma from some other primary site within the upper aerodigestive tract.
   ■ Branchial cyst is a possibility, although the lump is a little high and the patient a little too old.
   ■ Lymphomas frequently present as a lump in the neck.
   ■ An infective lymphadenopathy, e.g. TB or glandular fever.
   ■ A submandibular gland swelling, although this will usually give rise to a swelling under the ramus of the mandible.
3   Nasopharynx, oral cavity (tonsil, tongue and floor of mouth), larynx (especially the supraglottis), pyriform fossae, postcricoid region and upper oesophagus.

## Adenoid cystic carcinoma

This has nothing whatsoever to do with the adenoid. It is a tumour of minor salivary glands, arising wherever these glands are found. They often affect the nose and tend to spread along nerves (perineural infiltration). They rarely metastasize and the short-term prognosis is good. However, most patients will die from their disease within 10–20 years.

## T-cell lymphoma

Previously known as *lethal midline granuloma* and *Stewart's granuloma*, this has now been recognized as a true lymphoma. It causes massive destruction of the nose, face and sinuses, and is usually rapidly fatal. Treatment is with radiation.

## Nasopharyngeal carcinoma

The old name for this was *lymphoepithelioma*. This was misleading since it is in fact a variant of squamous cell carcinoma. It may cause no symptoms until a metastatic neck node is noted. Involvement of the eustachian tube may lead to a glue ear and pain or paraesthesia may develop as a result of trigeminal nerve involvement. The tumour is common in China and the Far East and the Epstein–Barr virus has been implicated in its aetiology. Thankfully, the tumour is radiosensitive since successful surgical excision in this region is difficult.

# GRANULOMATOUS AND NON-GRANULOMATOUS INFECTION

## Granulomatous inflammation/infection

### Wegener's granulomatosis

This is a systemic condition of unknown aetiology which is characterized by perivascular non-caseating granulomatous inflammation. It can affect any part of the respiratory system (including the middle ear). In the nose it can present either with a septal perforation, a patch of ulceration or a raised abnormal-looking area. Wegener's granulomatosis is a multisystem disease and may affect the skin and joints. However, it is its renal and pulmonary effects which are potentially life-threatening. A raised erythrocyte sedimentation rate (ESR) and positive antinuclear cytoplasmic antibody (ANCA) test are suggestive of this condition, but a biopsy is usually diagnostic. Treatment is with high-dose steroids, cyclophosphamide and/or azathioprine. The ENT team should involve the help of a physician who has experience in the systemic effects of this condition, at an early stage.

## Sarcoidosis

This may cause nodules on, or within, the nose. Again it is a multisystem disease and may affect the salivary glands, skin and uveal tract. A raised serum angiotensin-converting enzyme (ACE) and biopsy are diagnostic.

## Syphilis and tuberculosis

These are infections characterized by granulomatous inflammation, both of which can affect the nose, leading to ulceration and septal perforation. Diagnosis and treatment are as for other forms of these diseases.

## Non-granulomatous infection

### Scleroma

This is rare in the UK and is due to a *Klebsiella* infection. There is formation of a tumour-like mass within the nasal cavity, which in time leads to progressive scarring and stenosis of the nasal cavity. The condition is treated with streptomycin.

### Aspergillosis

This is a fungal infection which causes a chronic, low-grade sinusitis. However, it can also behave as an aggressive potentially fatal infection in immunocompromised patients.

### Rhinosporidiosis

This is a fungal infection, most often seen in India. It presents as a bleeding polyp of the septum. It is spread from cow faeces and is treated with wide local excision.

---

**KEY POINTS**

**Tumours and Destructive Lesions of the Nose**

- A wide variety of different tumours may present with similar symptoms
- The most common symptoms of nasal tumours are unilateral nasal obstruction, blood-stained rhinorrhoea and a lump in the nose
- The most common benign nasal tumour is an inverted papilloma; the most common malignant is a squamous cell carcinoma
- Most of the non-neoplastic, destructive lesions of the nose lead to a raised ESR, but biopsy is usually required to confirm the diagnosis

---

# EPISTAXIS

This is a common problem, which will affect most of us at some time in our lives (see also pages 156–157). Usually it is mild and self-limiting. However, it can be life-threatening and is always a frightening experience for the patient. The commonest causes of epistaxis are nose-picking and idiopathic:

- Local causes
  - Idiopathic
  - Trauma
  - Infection
  - Tumours
- Systemic causes
  - Hypertension
  - Anticoagulant drugs
  - Coagulopathy
  - Hereditary haemorrhagic telangiectasia

Due to its rich blood supply and propensity for digital trauma, the anterior septum is the most frequent site of bleeding.

Hypertension alone, rarely causes a nose bleed but it is often an accompanying feature in severe cases since it will prolong bleeding, as will anticoagulant drugs such as warfarin. Non-steroidal anti-inflammatory drugs (NSAIDs) such as aspirin are also associated with epistaxis since these inhibit platelet function. Haematological diseases such as haemophilia and Von Willebrand's disease, as well as leukaemia and disseminated intravascular coagulation (DIC) can lead to nose bleeding.

One condition in particular deserves special mention. This is hereditary haemorrhagic telangiectasia (HHT). Here, multiple abnormal capillaries occur and may be found throughout the respiratory, gastrointestinal and urogenital tracts, as well as the skin. The most effective treatments consist in argon laser cautery of the telangectasias and closure of the nostril (Young's operation). Although poorly tolerated by many patients, this does dramatically reduce the number and severity of nose bleeds.

Unilateral, severe nose bleeds in an adolescent boy should alert one to the possibility of a juvenile angiofibroma (see page 135).

First-aid measures, assessment and management of an epistaxis are covered on pages 156–157. Severe epistaxis may require examination of the nose under anaesthesia, with diathermy, postnasal space packing or even ligation of the maxillary, anterior ethmoidal or external carotid arteries.

# RHINOPLASTY AND FACIAL PLASTIC SURGERY

Patients may request cosmetic facial surgery in order to reverse the effects of ageing or because they consider themselves unattractive. Patients must be selected for this surgery with extreme care as a percentage will have unstable personalities or may even be frankly

## KEY POINTS
### Epistaxis

- This is a common condition which usually responds to simple first-aid manoeuvres
- More severe bleeding primarily affects the elderly
- The commonest site is the anterior septum (Little's area)
- The commonest causes are idiopathic and nose-picking
- Prolonged bleeding is associated with hypertension, anticoagulants and NSAIDs
- Rarely, nasal tumours may present with an epistaxis

## CASE STUDY

Eddie is 72 years old and presents to the Accident & Emergency department with a severe left-sided nose bleed. It has been going on for 2 hours and shows no sign of abating. He has never had a nose bleed before and has no nasal problems. However, he did have a cold last week. Examination finds him bleeding briskly from the left side; his blood pressure is 190/130 and pulse 88.

1 What relevant points have been omitted from this history?
2 What investigations should you order?
3 How should he be managed?

### Comments

1 Relevant past medical history will include details of cardiovascular problems such as hypertension, cerebrovascular accident ('stroke'), heart failure, etc., as well as any history of haematological conditions, especially bleeding problems. The drug history is particularly important since many elderly patients take aspirin or other non-steroidal anti-inflammatory or other drugs which can prolong bleeding.
2 Full blood count (FBC), coagulation screen and group and save are the essential blood tests which should be ordered.
3 If the bleeding point can be identified then cautery may be applied. If this is not possible or unsuccessful, then he should have the nose packed and be admitted and confined to bed. Many ENT surgeons would advocate the use of prophylactic antibiotics and sedation when nasal packing is *in situ*. A rapid assessment of his blood loss and cardiovascular status must be performed and intravenous fluid replacement or blood transfusion commenced if necessary.

psychotic! The realistic results of surgery must be explained honestly in order to avoid disappointment. However, having given these warnings it must be said that the results from successful surgery can be most satisfying both for the patient and surgeon.

## Rhinoplasty

This is a cosmetic operation which aims to improve the aesthetic appearance of the nose. Septorhinoplasty will also attempt to improve the nasal airway by repositioning a deviated septum. Both the patient and the surgeon must be aware of the surgical priority: airway or appearance. Details of rhinoplasty are beyond the scope of this book, but we shall outline the most common negative features of the nose which rhinoplasty can improve.

- An overly large nose can be made smaller with a reduction rhinoplasty.
- Deviation of the nasal bones and/or deviation of the cartilaginous septum may be straightened with a septorhinoplasty.
- A broad nasal bridge may be narrowed.
- Nasal hump is a common feature after a nasal injury and may be removed.
- Dorsal saddling results from inadequate support for the dorsum of the nose, usually as a result of destruction of the dorsal cartilaginous septum. This may be augmented using cartilage, bone or a silastic prosthesis.
- Over- or under-rotation of the nasal tip can also be corrected.

## Pinnaplasty

This is performed for patients with prominent, or bat-ears. Usually there is poor development of the antihelical fold, which leads to ears which stick out, rather than actually being too big. This can be corrected with simple surgery to recreate this fold. Occasionally, there is overdevelopment of the conchal bowl and this needs to be corrected if a satisfactory result is to be achieved.

## Mentoplasty

This is performed if the chin is too big or too small. This may involve insertion of a prosthesis, or moving the mandible forward or backwards.

## Blepharoplasty

This involves excision of the excess skin and peri-orbital fat, which cause wrinkles and bags around the eyes. Facial wrinkles can be treated by collagen injection or the excess skin excised with a face lift.

# 11

# The paranasal sinuses

Structure and function of the sinuses  140

Sinusitis  142

Tumours of the sinuses  147

Facial trauma  148

This chapter should not be read in isolation, since much of the material covered in Chapter 10 concerning the nose and nasal cavities is relevant to the following text. We describe the nose and sinuses separately so as not to overload the reader with information. Hopefully, the reader will gain an understanding of the overall picture, piece by piece.

# STRUCTURE AND FUNCTION OF THE SINUSES

The sinuses are air-filled outpouchings of the nasal cavity which invaginate the bones of the skull. Their exact function remains uncertain. However, several reasons have been postulated for their existence. None of these has been proven:

- To reduce the weight of the skull.
- To increase the resonance of the voice.
- To protect the eye and brain from physical trauma, by acting rather like 'crumple zones' found in a motor car.
- To separate the nasal cavity and brain, and hence protect the cranial contents from cooling as a result of nasal air flow.

Anatomically, the sinuses are described in four pairs: frontal, ethmoid, maxillary and sphenoid (Figure 11.1). Each of these drains into the nasal cavity. The sinuses may be divided functionally into an anterior group and a posterior group, depending upon into which area of the nasal cavity they drain. The anterior group (the maxillary and anterior ethmoidal sinuses) drains into the middle meatus, under the middle turbinate. This area is known as the ostiomeatal unit (Figure 11.2) and is clinically highly significant. Occasionally pneumatisation of the middle turbinate (concha bullosa) occurs (Figure 11.3) and this may cause narrowing of the middle meatus and ostiomeatal complex. The posterior group (the posterior ethmoids and sphenoid sinuses) drains into the nasal cavity in the superior meatus or sphenoethmoidal recess (Figure 11.4).

The mucosa of the sinuses is similar in type to the rest of the nasal cavity and respiratory tract, i.e. ciliated columnar. Ciliary action is important in clearing secretions from the sinuses into the nasal cavity via small channels called ostia. Ciliary dysfunction may cause, as well as result from, sinusitis. Mucociliary clearance pathways have been demonstrated (Figure 11.5).

Each of the sinuses is closely related to important structures and as a result, these can become involved in diseases which affect the sinuses (Figure 11.6). The relationships between the sinuses are outlined in Table 11.1.

TABLE 11.1 Relations of the sinuses

| MAXILLARY | ETHMOID | SPHENOID | FRONTAL |
| --- | --- | --- | --- |
| Orbit | Orbit | Internal carotid | Orbit |
| Teeth | Cribriform plate | Cavernous sinus | Brain |
| Cheek | Optic nerve | Pituitary | |

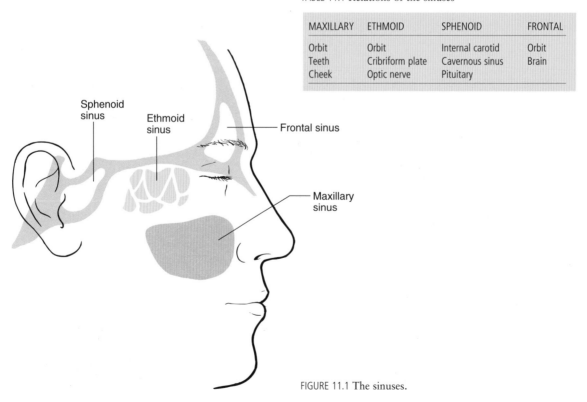

FIGURE 11.1 The sinuses.

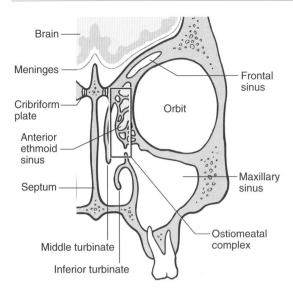

FIGURE 11.2 The ostiomeatal complex.

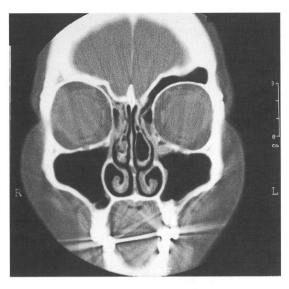

FIGURE 11.3 Pneumatization of the left middle turbinate, or concha bullosa.

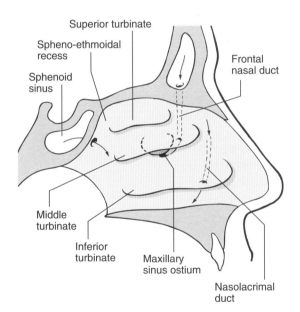

FIGURE 11.4 Drainage of the nasolacrimal duct and sinuses.

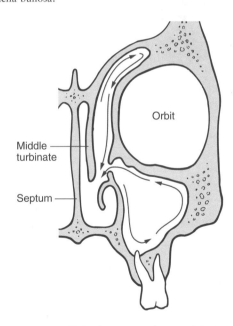

FIGURE 11.5 Mucociliary clearance pathways of the frontal and maxillary sinuses.

## KEY POINTS
### The Sinuses and Nasal Cavity

- The sinuses and nasal cavity must be considered together, both physiologically and pathologically
- The cranial cavity and the eye are both closely related to the sinuses and therefore may be involved in sinus disease and are potentially at risk during sinus surgery
- Most of the sinuses drain into the middle meatus. As a result, a small amount of congestion here can lead to widespread sinus dysfunction

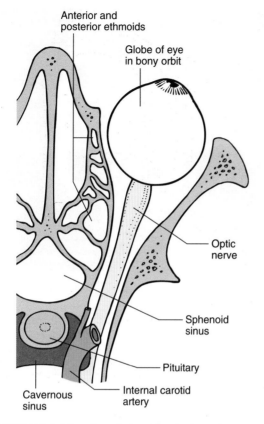

FIGURE 11.6 Axial section of ethmoid and sphenoid sinuses showing the important anatomical relationships.

# SINUSITIS

The symptoms of sinusitis can be classed as either acute or chronic:

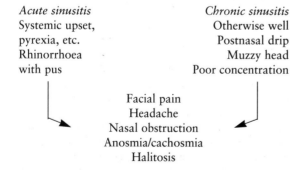

*Acute sinusitis*
Systemic upset, pyrexia, etc.
Rhinorrhoea with pus

*Chronic sinusitis*
Otherwise well
Postnasal drip
Muzzy head
Poor concentration

Facial pain
Headache
Nasal obstruction
Anosmia/cachosmia
Halitosis

## Acute sinusitis

Sinusitis is an inflammation of the lining of the sinuses. It is commonly infective in origin and usually results from a simple viral rhinosinusitis (the common

## OVERVIEW
### Diseases of the Sinuses

**Congenital**
■ Hypoplasia of a sinus

**Acquired**

**Trauma**
■ Direct trauma: facial fracture
■ **Eye trauma**: blow-out fracture
■ Head trauma: anterior skull-base fracture
■ **Barotrauma**

**Infection**
■ **Viral**, e.g. Rhinovirus
■ **Bacterial**, e.g. *Streptococcus*
■ **Fungal**, *e.g.* Aspergillus
■ Other, e.g. TB

**Tumours**
*Benign*
■ Squamous papilloma
■ **Inverted papilloma**
■ Osteoma
■ Fibrous dysplasia
■ **Angiofibroma**
*Malignant*
■ **Squamous cell carcinoma**
■ **Adenocarcinoma**
■ Malignant melanoma
■ T-cell lymphoma
■ Sarcomas

cold). This primary infection has the effects of reducing ciliary function, causing oedema of the nasal mucosa and sinus ostia and increasing nasal secretions. These stagnant secretions within the sinuses may become secondarily infected by bacteria, commonly *Streptococcus* or *Haemophilus*.

Certain conditions may predispose to sinusitis. These include any condition which blocks the ostia of the sinuses, such as nasal polyps, or conditions which interfere with air flow through the nose, for example a deviated septum. The roots of the upper teeth often project into the maxillary sinus and thus dental infections can also lead to sinusitis. The diagnosis of acute sinusitis is usually made on the clinical history and examination. Sinus X-rays are confirmatory, but generally computed tomography scans of the sinuses give

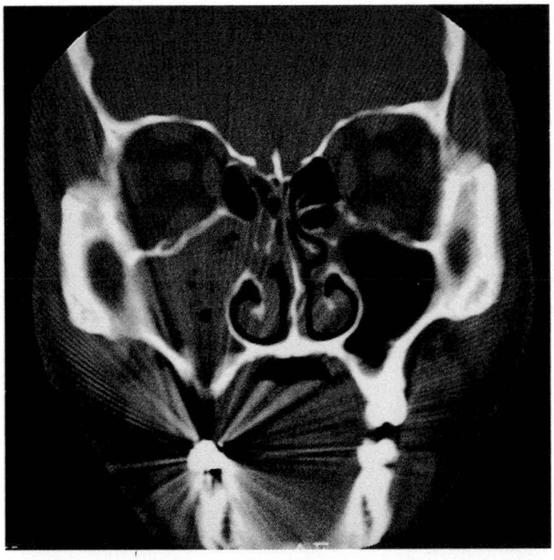

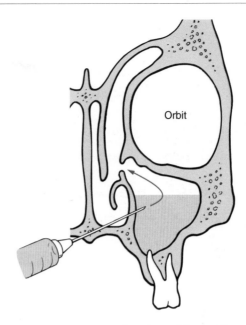

FIGURE 11.9 Aspiration and washout of the maxillary antrum.

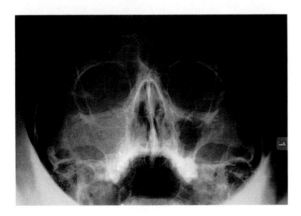

FIGURE 11.7 Right maxillary sinusitis occurring as a result of dental infection. Note the anatomical details and extent of disease which are well demonstrated with computed tomography (CT) scanning.

FIGURE 11.8 Right maxillary sinusitis as seen on X-ray (compare to Figure 11.7, showing a CT of the same patient).

far more information, and show the exact extent of the disease (Figures 11.7 and 11.8).

## Treatment of acute sinusitus

The main aim of treatment in acute sinusitis is to reduce inflammation of the sinus ostia using topical nasal decongestants such as ephedrine and also to combat bacterial infection with antibiotics. Analgesics such as paracetamol are usually required in addition. In cases which fail to resolve with the above treatment, or where complications are apparent, aspiration

and washout of the maxillary antrum (Figure 11.9) will usually speed recovery.

## Complications of acute sinusitis

These include:

- Chronic sinusitis
- Facial cellulitis
- Peri-orbital cellulitis
- Osteomyelitis
- Meningitis
- Brain abscess
- Mucocoele formation

### Acute frontal sinusitis

Acute frontal sinusitis deserves special mention, since it is important to recognize and treat this condition early in order to avoid the life- and sight-threatening complications which can occur with infections of this sinus. It presents as tenderness over the forehead, especially on percussion. Severe frontal headache, becoming worse on bending, is characteristic. The infection can easily spread to the orbit where blindness can occur with little warning. Another danger of frontal sinusitis is the spread of infection to the cranial cavity, with formation of an extradural or intracranial abscess (Figure 11.10). Patients with frontal sinusitis should be treated aggressively, with broad-spectrum antibiotics and decongestants. However, if there is any

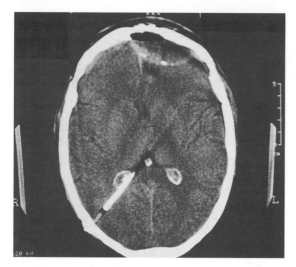

FIGURE 11.10 A CT scan of a patient with an extradural frontal abscess resulting from frontal sinusitis. Note also the intraventricular shunt required due to the raised intracranial pressure.

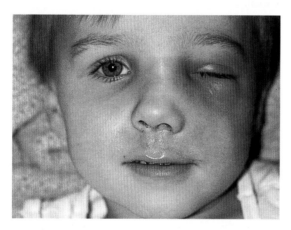

FIGURE 11.11 Peri-orbital cellulitis arising as a consequence of ethmoidal sinusitis.

## CASE STUDY

Jackie is 44 years old and presents to the Accident & Emergency department complaining of a hot, red, painful swollen left eye for the past 12 hours. She had a cold last week and also complains of a frontal headache. Examination shows the eye to be completely closed due to great swelling of the eyelids and peri-orbital tissues. She does not complain of any visual disturbance.

1 Which department should this patient be referred to and why?
2 Why is this a dangerous condition?
3 What are the important eye signs?
4 What is the essential investigation?

### Comments

1 This patient must be referred to the ENT department, since peri-orbital cellulitis is most often a complication of fronto-ethmoidal sinusitis. Moreover, if surgical intervention is required, the root cause of the infection must also be attended to if the condition is to resolve.
2 Preseptal peri-orbital cellulitis, i.e. infection limited to anterior to the tarsal plate, usually resolves quickly. However, the infection can easily spread to involve the orbit proper and intra-orbital infection can lead to optic nerve damage and blindness, often with alarming speed and with few warning signs.
3 Loss of colour vision, pain on eye movements, limitation of eye movements, diplopia and proptosis are suggestive of orbital involvement.
4 Computed tomography scanning of the sinuses will confirm the cause of the infection and is mandatory if there is any suggestion of orbital involvement.

complication at presentation, or if they are slow to show signs of recovery, surgical intervention, with drainage of the infected sinuses, is mandatory.

### Peri-orbital cellulitis

This may also be the presenting feature in ethmoidal sinus infection (Figure 11.11). It should be emphasized that this infection nearly always spreads from the sinuses and the patient must be referred to the ENT team, rather than the ophthalmologist. In such a case, the eye movements, visual acuity and colour vision must be checked, and if any defect is found, a computer tomography (CT) scan should be organized.

This will demonstrate any intra-orbital abscess. If present any intra-orbital pus must be drained at once.

### Mucocoeles

These usually form as late a complication of an acute sinusitis. They are collections of sterile mucus occupying an obstructed sinus (most commonly the frontal and ethmoidal). Over years, the sinus is expanded by mucus which is trapped under pressure within it. Because this is a slow process, it is usually asymptomatic until either the mucocoele becomes secondarily infected or the patient complains of facial swelling or develops visual problems as a result of displacement of the eye. Treatment is by surgical drainage of the sinus.

# Chronic sinusitis

The term 'chronic rhino-sinusitis' describes this condition more accurately since it occurs as a result of chronic nasal mucosal inflammation which is commonly infective, or allergic in origin. In fact, frequently a combination of infection and allergy is found.

Such long-standing mucosal inflammation induces cystic or polypoid changes in the lining of the nose and sinuses. The swollen mucosa further narrows the sinus ostia and so a vicious cycle results.

Medical treatment is initially aimed at the primary cause, infection and/or allergy, and entails the use of topical steroids and/or antibiotics. If this fails to resolve the condition, surgery may be required in order to improve sinus drainage.

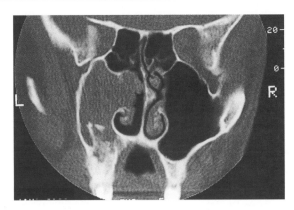

FIGURE 11.12 Maxillary fungal sinusitis; note the calcification within the sinus.

## Fungal sinusitis

This is rare and usually occurs in immunosupressed patients. It may follow an indolent course, e.g. as a result of Aspergillus infection, and the maxillary sinus is commonly infected; calcification is a common finding on CT (Figure 11.12). Even more uncommonly the disease may be fulminant and highly aggressive, in which case the mortality rate is high.

## Surgery for sinusitis

The basic aim of surgery is to improve drainage and hence increase aeration of the sinuses. This may involve simple flushing, enlargement of the natural ostium, creation of an artificial drainage opening or even complete opening of the sinus into the nasal cavity.

Operations may be performed either via an external approach, with access via a skin incision on the face (Figure 11.13) or they can be performed via the nose. External operations are generally safer since they allow good access and identification of important structures such as the orbit, but by definition, entail scarring of the face. Pernasal operations can be performed with or without the aid of endoscopes. Fibreoptic endoscopes improve illumination and identification of important landmarks within the nasal cavity and so allow safe surgery to be performed in otherwise potentially hazardous areas.

In recent years, the trend has been towards endoscopic sinus surgery, which has been aimed at the middle meatus. This is termed 'functional endoscopic sinus surgery' or 'FESS'. The idea behind this approach is that by relieving middle meatal congestion, sinus inflammation will resolve naturally. Which type of surgical technique is employed depends on the sinus involved and extent of the disease, as well as the surgeon's preference.

### Maxillary antrum

*Antral aspiration and washout*, sometimes known as 'proof puncture', is used to confirm the diagnosis and aims to restore normal mucociliary clearance.

*Antrostomy* involves making a drainage hole into the sinus, usually the maxillary antrum. This may be an artificial hole (made in the inferior meatus) or may involve enlarging the natural sinus ostium (in the middle meatus). Nowadays, this is usually performed with the aid of an endoscope.

The *Caldwell–Luc operation* involves removal of the diseased mucosal lining of the maxillary sinus. It is performed via a sublabial incision with removal of the anterior wall of the sinus. As part of the procedure, an antrostomy is also performed. Diagnostic endoscopic antroscopy can also be performed via a sublabial approach.

### Ethmoid sinuses

These are a honeycomb of air cells, separated by very thin bone. There is no single ostium, but instead multiple tiny openings into the nasal cavity. Therefore, operations to improve drainage of the ethmoid must involve the opening of these air cells into the nasal cavity with breaking down of the thin bony septae between each chamber. This can be performed via an external or an intranasal approach.

### Frontal sinus

*Trephination* (drilling a hole) in the floor of the frontal sinus is used to decompress an infected sinus.

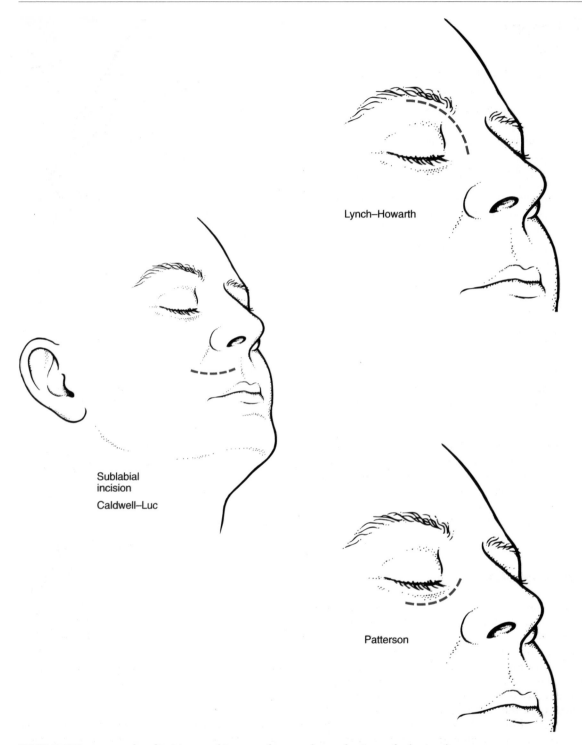

Lynch–Howarth

Sublabial
incision

Caldwell–Luc

Patterson

FIGURE 11.13 Some examples of incisions used in external approaches to the sinuses for benign disease.

Fronto-ethmoidectomy is required to drain the frontal sinus into the nasal cavity and involves removal of the floor of the frontal sinus and the eth- moid. The frontal sinus is difficult to access via the nose, and this operation is usually performed via an external approach.

## KEY POINTS
### Sinusitis

- Conditions such as nasal polyposis and upper-jaw dental infection may predispose to sinusitis
- Acute sinusitis is treated with nasal decongestants and antibiotics
- Beware acute frontal sinusitis – the complications may threaten sight or life
- Peri-orbital cellulitis usually results from sinus infection
- Medical treatment for chronic sinusitis usually consists of topical steroids with or without antibiotics
- Sinus surgery aims to allow the sinuses to drain and increase aeration. This may be performed pernasally or via an external approach

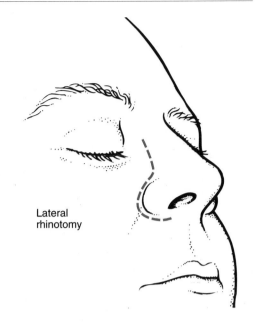

Lateral rhinotomy

# TUMOURS OF THE SINUSES

The same tumours which affect the nasal cavity affect the sinuses and much of the detail of these tumours has already been discussed in Chapter 10. This will not be repeated here. Suffice it to say that tumours of the sinuses usually present with nasal obstruction, unilateral nasal discharge (which is often blood-stained) or with frank epistaxis. Other symptoms which suggest extension beyond the confines of the sinuses include facial swelling, proptosis, pain or a metastatic deposit in a neck node.

## Treatment of sinus tumours

### Surgical excision

This may be achieved intranasally for small, benign tumours. On the whole, however, external approaches are preferred (Figure 11.14). The site and size of malignant tumours will determine the necessary extent of resection. For example, a large tumour arising from the maxillary sinus and invading the orbit may require radical maxillectomy and exenteration of the orbital contents. In radical maxillectomy, the hard palate is removed and the resulting defect filled with a dental prosthesis called an obturator (Figure 11.15). This serves to fill out the cheek as well as dividing the nasal and oral cavities. This is necessary for effective eating, drinking and talking. When the eye is removed, a prosthetic eye, which may be mounted on osseo-integrated implants, frequently gives a very satisfactory cosmetic result.

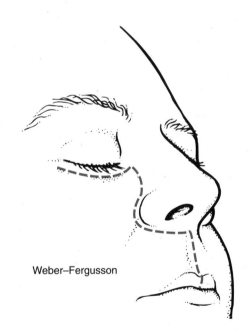

Weber–Fergusson

FIGURE 11.14 Some examples of incisions used for external approaches to the sinuses for sinus tumours.

Tumours which occupy the roof of the nose, and abut or invade the anterior skull base require *craniofacial resection*.

### Radiotherapy

Radiotherapy is used in appropriate cases, either as the primary treatment or in conjunction with surgery.

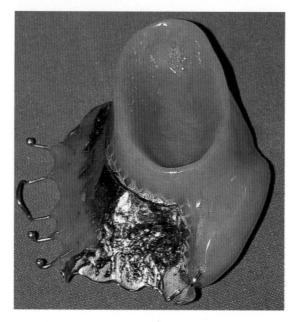

FIGURE 11.15 An obturator for use in a patient after maxillectomy.

Close liaison with the oncologist and radiotherapist, usually in a joint clinic, is essential when dealing with these cases.

# FACIAL TRAUMA

## Soft-tissue trauma

Due to the excellent blood supply of the face, soft-tissue wounds to the face will usually heal well. Facial lacerations should be accurately repaired with fine non-absorbable sutures which should be removed after 5 days. Extensive or complex wounds should be explored in order to exclude damage to important neurovascular structures.

## Facial fractures

### Nasal fractures

These are discussed in Chapter 10.

### Fractures of the zygoma (cheekbone) (Figure 11.16a)

These are usually caused by direct trauma to the cheek. Soon after the injury, the depression of the

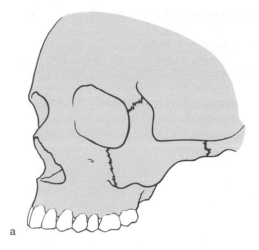

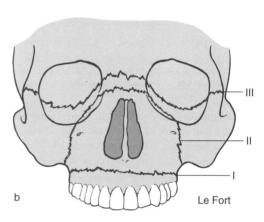

FIGURE 11.16 Facial fractures. (a) Zygoma; (b) maxillary (Le Fort Types I, II and III are shown).

cheek which results may be apparent. However, swelling of the overlying soft tissues rapidly obscures this defect, and the diagnosis should be suspected if there is bony tenderness or a step is palpable in the bone. Numbness over the cheek indicates that the infra-orbital nerve has been damaged. Elevation of the depressed segment is achieved via an inscision within the hairline.

### Maxillary fractures (Figure 11.16b)

Le Fort described three types of fractures of the maxilla. A large degree of trauma is associated with these fractures and other injuries should be sought. However, the immediate threat to life is usually due to obstruction to the airway and/or bleeding at the fracture site. The jaw and maxilla must be held forward in order to reduce these risks. These fractures require fixation for several weeks.

## Orbital blow-out fracture

This is caused by direct anterior trauma to the eyeball which is forced into the bony orbit. The increase in pressure within the orbit leads to a fracture in its weak floor. Some of the contents of the orbit, fat or the inferior rectus muscle may then prolapse into the maxillary sinus. This is well seen on X-ray or computed tomography and leads to enophthalmos and restriction of eye movements. Release of the tethered tissue and repair of the bony defect are required.

## Cerebrospinal fluid (CSF) rhinorrhoea

This occasionally occurs spontaneously, but more often complicates trauma to the skull, especially in the region of the cribriform plate or posterior wall of the frontal sinus. The patient will complain of crystal-clear watery rhinorrhoea. This can be diagnosed by testing positive for glucose or β-transferrin. The obvious danger is that the patient may develop an ascending meningitis and many ENT surgeons would give prophylactic antibiotics. A computed tomography scan of the area may confirm the defect and at operation the leak may be identified in the nose by observing a trickle of fluorescein which has been previously injected into the epidural space.

### KEY POINTS
Facial Trauma

- Secure the airway
- Control haemorrhage
- Consider other associated injury, e.g. cervical spine and head injury; treat these appropriately
- Fractures of the zygoma and orbital blow-out fractures are frequently missed; remember them and X-ray appropriately
- Watery anterior rhinorrhoea suggests a CSF leak; this may be confirmed by testing the fluid for glucose with a dip stick

# 12

# The ENT manifestations of AIDS and HIV infection

Sites where infection is manifested  152

HIV tests and counselling  153

How to protect yourself  153

The acquired immunodeficiency syndrome (AIDS) is one of the most significant diseases to have been recognized in the last century. It has had a widespread effect on all branches of clinical medicine, not least ENT. Despite massive research efforts, this is a universally fatal disease whose prevalence is increasing year on year. Head and neck manifestations of AIDS are common. In fact between 40 and 70% of all AIDS patients will initially present with symptoms in this area. It is vital that ENT surgeons are aware of the manifestations of AIDS in order that they may correctly diagnose and manage these patients, as well as take appropriate steps to prevent infection of themselves or those in their team. In the UK and the USA, AIDS is still principally a disease of sexually active homosexual men and intravenous drug abusers. However, more recently there has been a slight increase in affected heterosexual men and women. Prior to the current rigorous controls affecting blood products, haemophiliacs were at risk from the use of pooled factor VIII.

HIV primarily affects T-helper cells, which are central to cell-mediated immunity. Affected patients are therefore susceptible to a variety of opportunistic infections including mycobacterial, viral and fungal. Certain malignancies are also more common in AIDS patients.

## SITES WHERE INFECTION IS MANIFESTED

### The mouth

This is probably the most commonly affected site, particularly at the onset of AIDS. Kaposi's sarcoma (Figure 12.1) is a common lesion in AIDS patients and may affect any part of the skin and mucosal surfaces in the gastrointestinal tract, particularly the palate, gum and posterior pharyngeal wall. Oral candidiasis is also common, and may either present as an adherent white membrane or a red mucosal surface. If the diagnosis is in any doubt, one should take scrapings from the affected mucosa and submit them for microbiological analysis.

Herpes simplex infections are common in AIDS patients and cause mucosal ulcers which may vary from a few millimetres to several centimetres in size. Hairy leukoplakia (Figure 12.2) (named as a result of its histological appearance) of the tongue gives rise to characteristic appearance and only occurs in AIDS patients.

Deposits of non-Hodgkin's lymphoma may affect the mouth, particularly the tonsil.

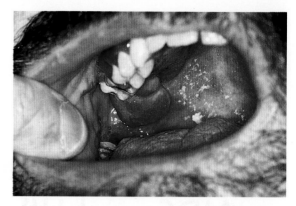

FIGURE 12.1 Kaposi's sarcoma of mouth. Published with the kind permission of Dr Lewis, St George's Hospital, London.

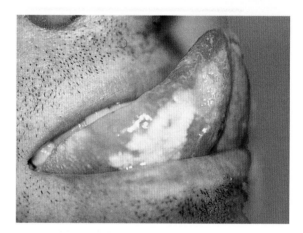

FIGURE 12.2 Hairy leukoplakia. Published with the kind permission of Dr Hay, St George's Hospital, London.

### The larynx

Epiglottitis and supraglottitis are not limited to those infected with HIV. However, AIDS patients are more susceptible to these and other serious infections. Intervention may be required in order to secure the airway. Kaposi's sarcoma of the larynx has also been reported.

### The nose and sinuses

Acute or chronic infections of the nose and sinuses are extremely common in AIDS and present with the usual symptoms of rhinorrhoea, postnasal drip, nasal obstruction, facial pain and headaches. In some cases, the causative agents are similar to those seen in patients without AIDS. However, unusual pathogens within the nose and sinuses may also be encountered, e.g. fungi, cytomegalovirus, Cryptococcus and even maggots! Once more, Kaposi's sarcoma and lymphomas may affect the nose, sinuses and nasopharynx.

## The ear

Otitis media (acute and chronic) and otitis externa are also common in AIDS patients. Again, these conditions may be due to the usual infective agents or in some cases due to less common organisms such as *Pneumocystis* causing otitis externa. The development of a unilateral glue ear must alert one to the possibility of a nasopharyngeal neoplasm obstructing the eustachian tube. Also, hearing loss may occur either as a result of infection of the auditory nerve directly, or as a sequelae of meningitis.

## The salivary glands

Dry mouth is a common complaint amongst HIV-infected patients. The precise cause remains uncertain; treatment is symptomatic. Parotid gland enlargement is common and may be uni- or bilateral. Such enlargement is unusual in that it has a cystic nature and these are evident on computed tomography or magnetic resonance imaging scanning. Surgery is best avoided and simple aspiration, repeated as necessary, is often sufficient to control symptoms.

## Neck nodes

One of the earliest recognized manifestations of HIV infection was persistent generalized lymphadenopathy (PGL). This is defined as the presence of nodes at least 1 cm in diameter, present at two extra-inguinal sites for three months or more. In this case, the nodes are symmetrical, mobile and non-tender. Other causes of cervical lymphadenopathy include lymphomas and Kaposi's sarcoma.

## Lower respiratory tree

Cough, shortness of breath and a low-grade fever may occur with infection of the bronchopulmonary tract. Pneumonia in AIDS patients is most commonly a result of *Pneumocystis carinii* but can also occur with *Cryptococcus*, *Histoplasma* and *Candida* infections.

# HIV TESTS AND COUNSELLING

If a patient is suspected of having HIV infection, their consent should be obtained prior to an HIV test being performed. Also, they must be counselled appropriately, preferably by experienced staff in either the infectious diseases or genitourinary departments.

# HOW TO PROTECT YOURSELF

- When dealing with any known or suspected HIV-positive patient, all healthcare workers should take appropriate precautions to prevent transmission via a transcutaneous or transmucosal route.
- Appropriate barrier precautions should be used to prevent skin and mucous membranes coming into contact with blood or body fluids, e.g. saliva, cerumen and tears. This will usually consist of gloves, with goggles and a mask when performing invasive procedures.
- Needles, scalpels and other sharp instruments should be used with great care. Needles should not be recapped or bent, and scalpels should not be passed from hand to hand.
- Healthcare workers with broken skin or weeping dermatitis should refrain from direct patient contact.

## CASE STUDY

John is brought into casualty unconscious. He is in his twenties and extremely unkempt. He is well known to the staff in the department as an intravenous drug abuser and is suspected of having taken a drug overdose. On examination, he is noted to have several neck swellings which are soft and isolated from one another, they are approximately symmetrical. Examination of his mouth shows a dark brown, raised lesion 1 cm × 1 cm on his hard palate. His hospital records show that he is a frequent attender with drugs-related problems; however, recently he has also presented with two bouts of tonsillitis and one ear infection.

1  What is the diagnosis?
2  What extra precautions should be taken by the hospital staff?

**Comments**

1  It is very likely that he has AIDS. Persistent generalized lymphadenopathy (PGL) in combination with oral Kaposi's sarcoma on a background of frequent infections make the diagnosis almost beyond doubt.

2  All staff should take precautions to avoid contact with blood products and body fluids of any patient. However, in this case one should be especially careful when taking blood and handling sharps. All samples must be labelled as 'high risk' in order to warn the laboratory staff of the increased risk.

# 13

# Procedures in ENT

How to stop a nose bleed (epistaxis)  156
How to remove foreign bodies  157
How to syringe an ear  160
How to mop an ear  160

How to drain a haematoma of the pinna (haematoma auris)  161
How to drain a quinsy  161

# HOW TO STOP A NOSE BLEED (EPISTAXIS)

## Provoking factors

From the history, consider these provoking factors, and where possible correct them:

■ Trauma
■ Hypertension
■ (NSAIDs) Anticoagulants
■ Upper respiratory tract infections
■ Clotting disorder

## First aid (Figure 13.1)

■ Lean forward
■ Pinch the fleshy part of the nose (not the bridge) for 10 min
■ Avoid swallowing the blood
■ Ice pack on the nasal bridge

## Resuscitation

Resuscitate in cases of severe epistaxis.

■ Assess blood loss
■ Pulse
■ Blood pressure
■ Gain intravenous access
■ Set up an intravenous infusion if the blood loss is great or there is cardiovascular compromise
■ Full blood count
■ Coagulation
■ Group and save

## Further management

■ Use a thudicums speculum or auroscope to examine Little's area (anterior part of the septum). This is most often the site of bleeding.
■ If a bleeding point is seen, spray the nose with 5% cocaine, xylocaine or another topical local anaesthetic and attempt nasal cautery. If the bleeding is severe and no bleeding point is seen, then the nose will need to be packed.

## How to cauterize the nose

■ Apply one or two cotton buds or a dental roll soaked in 1:200 000 adrenaline or 5% cocaine solution to the area and apply pressure for at least 2 min.

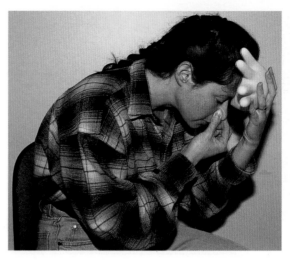

FIGURE 13.1 The position which should be adopted in patients with an epistaxis. A rubber glove can be filled with ice and applied to the nasal bridge/forehead.

■ Use silver nitrate cautery sticks which should be applied for 1–2 s at a time. Start a few millimetres from the bleeding point, working in a circle, to cauterize any *feeder* blood vessels before attempting to cauterize the main bleeding point.
■ Most anterior nose bleeds can be cauterized successfully with skill and patience. Often you will need to re-apply the adrenaline or cocaine as above in order to reduce the blood flow between attempts at cautery.
■ If unsuccessful, then re-apply pressure to stem the flow and pack the nose.

## How to pack the nose

When the bleeding point is posterior and therefore not easily accessible for cautery, or when cautery has failed, the nose will need to be packed. The idea is to put pressure onto the bleeding vessel to prevent active haemorrhage so that the normal thrombotic mechanisms can act. Nasal packs are usually left in place for 24–48 hours. They must be secured anteriorly to prevent them prolapsing backwards into the airway. Most ENT departments give prophylactic antibiotics whilst packing is in place. Having the nose packed is uncomfortable and can interfere with the patient's breathing. For these reasons, most patients who require nasal packs are admitted to hospital and lightly sedated. Nasal packs may be placed anteriorly, posteriorly or both. They may also be unilateral or bilateral. A variety of differing materials can be used to pack the nasal cavity. Those most commonly used are described below.

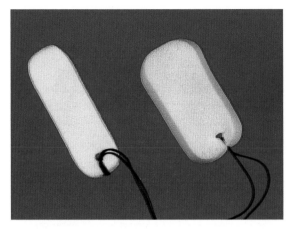

FIGURE 13.2 Nasal tampons before and after inflation with water.

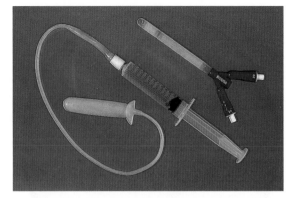

FIGURE 13.3 Two different types of epistaxis balloons, each with ports to allow inflation once correctly placed in the nose.

### Nasal tampons

Nasal tampons (Figure 13.2) are the simplest way to pack the nose. There is a number of these packs available today. They all consist of a desiccated, compressed sponge which when inflated with any water-based fluid, expands dramatically. They look a little bit like a lollypop stick when dry and require lubrication before insertion using Naseptin® cream. Lift the tip of the nose and slide the tampon into the nasal cavity, ensuring that it is passed parallel to the floor of the nose. It may then be inflated with water or saline and secured with a stitch passed through the tampon which is then taped to the face. The advantage of this form of packing is that effective haemostasis is usually achieved and no other equipment is required at all.

### BIPP (bismuth iodine and paraffin paste)

This is the traditional material used to pack the nose. It consists of a length of ribbon gauze which is impregnated with a mixture of antiseptics. This is effective if properly inserted but requires considerable skill to place correctly and is becoming less popular because it causes quite marked trauma to the nasal lining. Good lighting is essential. A thudicums speculum is inserted and the gauze is placed in a layered fashion into the nasal cavity using Tilley's dressing forceps. Topical analgesia, e.g. xylocaine or cocaine spray, is essential.

### Kaltostat

This is an alginate-based material which is packed into the nose under direct vision, similar to BIPP. It has some haemostaic potential of its own.

### Epistaxis balloon or Foley urinary catheter

There is a variety of specially designed nasal balloons available (Figure 13.3). They are simple to insert and are particularly useful when the bleeding point is posterior. They are placed into the nasal cavity and inflated. If necessary, an anterior pack can also be inserted. A Foley urinary catheter is also effective for posterior bleeds. Here, the catheter is passed to the nasopharynx, inflated and then pulled anteriorly so that it lodges in the posterior choana. Its position is maintained by using a clamp at the nasal vestibule. This must be cushioned in order to prevent pressure necrosis of the nasal inlet. An anterior pack is frequently also required with this method.

In all cases pack the side which is actively bleeding first, if bleeding continues pack the other side as well, this splints the septum and may achieve haemostasis.

## Referral policy

Indications for immediate referral are:

- Failure to control bleeding
- Need for resuscitation
- If the nose has been packed

Indications for late referral are:

- Recurrent small bleeds
- Unable to cauterize

# HOW TO REMOVE FOREIGN BODIES

## General principles

A good light source, a cooperative or well-restrained patient and the correct equipment are all essential for

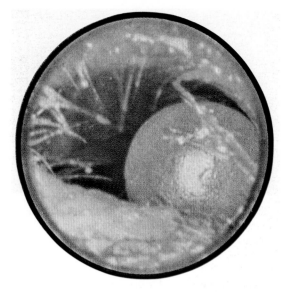

FIGURE 13.4 Bead in the ear.

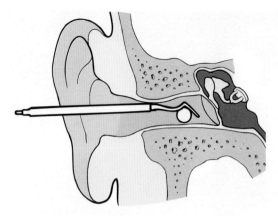

FIGURE 13.5 How to remove a foreign body from the ear.

the successful removal of foreign bodies in ENT practice. Most patients are children and here the first attempt is usually the most well tolerated. Therefore, if you are not confident that you will be able to remove the object, refer the patient to the ENT department.

## Foreign bodies in the ear (Figure 13.4)

The following are features which may accompany foreign bodies in the ear:

■ Unilateral discharge
■ Bleeding
■ Deafness
■ Pain

### Management

Most children, unless they are extremely cooperative, will require a general anaesthetic to remove the object. In adults, more often than not, foreign bodies can be removed without sedation. How the object is best removed will depend on the exact nature of the foreign body and the degree of trauma to the ear canal:

■ Insects may be drowned with olive oil.
■ Syringing may be used if there is no trauma to the eardrum or canal.
■ When removing a foreign body using an operating auroscope, head lamp or operating microscope remember that:

if the foreign body is soft, e.g. cotton wool, use crocodile, Tilley's or other grasping forceps; and if the foreign body is solid, e.g. a bead, then use a hook or Jobson horn probe to pass beyond the foreign body and gently pull towards you (Figure 13.5).

## Referral policy

■ Failed attempt at removal
■ Nearly always 'non-urgent'
■ Uncooperative children
■ Suspected trauma to eardrum
■ If there is a risk of damaging the eardrum during removal, then refer

## Foreign bodies in the nose

The following features may accompany a foreign body in the nose:

■ Unilateral foul-smelling nasal discharge (Figure 13.6)
■ Unilateral nasal obstruction
■ Unilateral vestibulitis
■ Epistaxis

### Management

■ Ask child to blow nose, if able.
■ As in the ear, if the foreign body is soft or has a thin free edge, then it may be grasped and removed with crocodile or Tilley's forceps. If it is solid and round, then it is best removed using a Jobson horn probe which has been bent slightly at the tip. Pass the

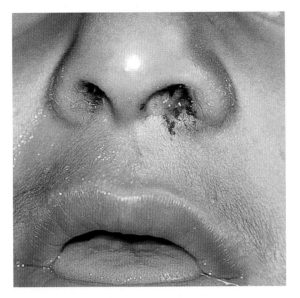

FIGURE 13.6 Foreign body in the nose.

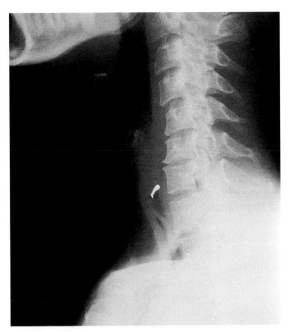

FIGURE 13.7 A metallic foreign body in the throat. Note also the abnormal straightness of the cervical spine indicating irritation and spasm of the prevertebral musculature.

probe beyond the foreign body and draw slowly towards you. Always check for a second foreign body.
■ An auroscope is often best for examining a child's nose.

## Complications

■ Vestibulitis
■ Inhalation of the foreign body

## Referral policy

Due to the potential risk of inhalation, all foreign bodies in the nose should be removed as soon as possible.

## Foreign bodies in the throat

A carefully taken history will often give the diagnosis. Features of oropharyngeal foreign bodies include:

■ Symptoms which usually come on straight away with a genuine foreign body, not a few hours or days later.
■ Bones, usually fish, chicken or lamb.
■ Pricking sensation or pain on every swallow.
■ Dysphagia.
■ Drooling.
■ Stridor (rare).
■ Point tenderness in the neck is suggestive as is pain on gently rocking the larynx from side to side.

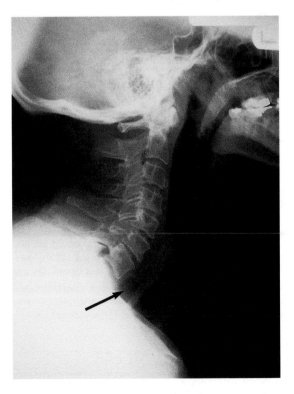

FIGURE 13.8 Air in the upper oesophagus – a sign of an impacted foreign body.

- If the patient localizes to above the thyroid cartilage, especially to one side, look carefully at the tongue base and tonsil.
- Perform lateral soft tissue X-rays of the neck (Figure 13.7) and look for foreign bodies at the common sites, i.e. tongue base and posterior pharyngeal wall; soft-tissue swelling alone is suggestive. Air in the upper oesophagus is suggestive of an oesophageal foreign body (Figure 13.8). Remember that small flecks of calcification around the thyroid and cricoid cartilages are quite common.

## Management

- Good light source (torch or head mirror).
- Use xylocaine spray to anaesthetise the throat.
- Use your finger to see if you can feel a foreign body, even if you cannot see one.
- Use Tilley's forceps for foreign bodies in the mouth or tonsil.
- Use McGill intubating forceps for foreign bodies in the tongue base or pharynx. Here, lie the patient flat, extend the neck and use an intubating laryngoscope to lift the tongue forward.

## Complications

- There is potential for inflammation/infection around an impacted foreign body leading to abscess formation or perforation of the oesophagus.
- Acute airway problem.

## Referral policy

- Any airway compromise should be referred at once. Otherwise, patients should be seen within 6 hours if:
- Failed attempt at removal
- Good history, but no foreign body seen
- X-ray evidence of a foreign body

In these circumstances rigid endoscopy under general anaesthesia may be indicated. This should be performed by an experienced ENT surgeon. Remember to keep patients nil by mouth in case a general anaesthetic is required.

# HOW TO SYRINGE AN EAR

Ear syringing is used to remove wax from the ear canal. Prior to performing this procedure, ensure that there is no previous history of tympanic membrane perforation, grommet insertion or ear surgery.

- Warm the water to body temperature.
- Pull the pinna upwards and backwards in order to straighten the ear canal.
- Using an ear syringe, aim the jet of water towards the roof of the ear canal.
- If the patient complains of pain at any point then *stop*.

# HOW TO MOP AN EAR

Any ear which is discharging purulent material will require aural toilet and treatment with combination antibiotic and steroid drops with or without oral antibiotics. The most common conditions which cause such a discharge are otitis externa and chronic suppurative otitis media (CSOM).

Aural toilet can most simply be performed by the patient, or relative, at home once they have been instructed correctly. Removing a large amount of the debris from the ear canal will speed resolution and will also allow better entry of the topical agents into the ear. The use of commercial cotton buds should be discouraged since they are both too traumatic and poorly absorbent. Instead, ear mops should be made in the following way.

A piece of clean cotton wool should be teased out into a flat sheet and then twisted onto a suitable carrier such as a Jobson–Horne probe, orange stick or even a clean matchstick. If constructed correctly this should be soft, highly absorbent and atraumatic (Figure 13.9). This is then inserted gently into the ear canal, having lifted the pinna upwards and backwards. The mop is gently rotated in the ear and then removed. This procedure is repeated until the cotton wool returns clean. Now the drops can be inserted. These should be instilled into the ear, with the patient lying

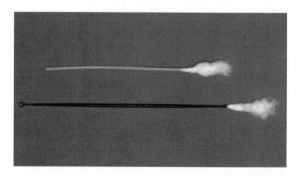

FIGURE 13.9 Ear mops which are easy to construct and have soft, absorbent, non-traumatic tips.

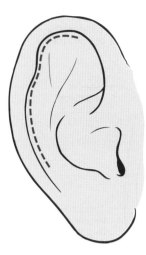

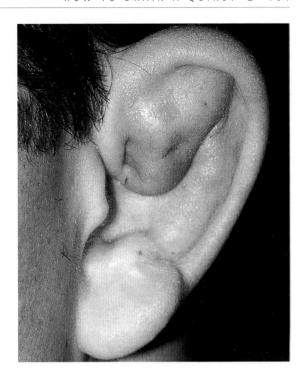

FIGURE 13.10 Incision of the skin of the pinna when draining a haematoma.

with the affected ear uppermost. The pinna should be gently moved backwards and forwards and the tragus massaged in order to encourage the drops to seep right down to the eardrum. After a few minutes, when the patient stands up, they will surely notice some of the drops running out of the ear. However, some will remain to be effective within the ear. 'Pope otowicks' are also often helpful in such patients. These are tiny sponge dressings, similar to the nasal tampons described above. When inflated with the drops, they expand and help to splint open an oedematous ear canal as well as acting as a reservoir for the drops. They should be removed/changed after 2–3 days.

## HOW TO DRAIN A HAEMATOMA OF THE PINNA (HAEMATOMA AURIS)

This follows direct trauma to the external ear and is common in sports injuries. A fluctuant purple swelling of the pinna follows. Delayed drainage of the haematoma may lead to fibrosis and necrosis of the cartilage of the pinna. This leads to a permanent deformity of the ear (cauliflower ear).

### Management

- Aspiration usually fails and is best avoided.

- It is probably best to refer to ENT for open drainage in sterile conditions.
- Technique:
   Incise the skin of the pinna in the helical sulcus under local anaesthetic (Figure 13.10).
   Milk out the haematoma.
   Do not close the wound. Some ENT surgeons use a drain routinely.
   Either pack the contours of the pinna with cotton wool soaked in proflavine or saline or use a through-and-through matress suture tied over a bolster in order to encourage the skin to adhere to the underlying cartilage.
   Light pressure bandage should be applied for 5 days.
   Remember tetanus and antibiotic prophylaxis.

Remember that the patient must have received a significant blow to the head and may also require treatment for this.

## HOW TO DRAIN A QUINSY

A quinsy or peritonsillar abscess usually presents with the following features:

- Sore throat which is worse on one side
- Pyrexia
- Trismus

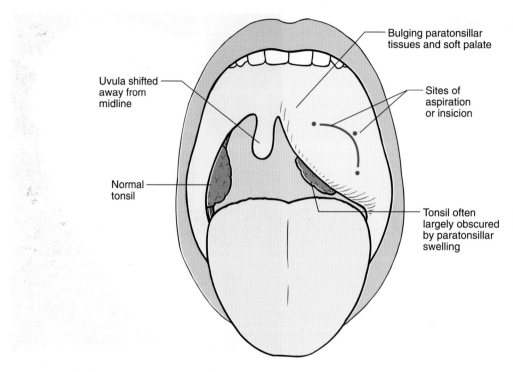

FIGURE 13.11 The characteristic appearance of a quinsy and suggested sites for aspiration/incision.

- Difficulty in swallowing or drooling
- Fetor
- Peritonsillar swelling on one side
- Displacement of the uvula away from the affected side

## Management

- These patients usually require admission for analgesia and rehydration.
- Antibiotics, intravenous if in hospital.
- Three-point aspiration or incision and drainage.

Drainage of the abscess cavity can be achieved by needle aspiration or incision. Personal preference usually decides which of these techniques is used. It is the author's practice to perform three-point aspiration initially and reserve incision for those cases which fail to resolve within 24 hours.

### Three-point aspiration

Anaesthesia is achieved either with topical sprays such as xyolcaine or with injected lignocaine. The patient is asked to lie on a couch and the procedure explained. Using a good light source, preferably a head light, a large bore needle (or intravenous cannula) attached to

a 10-ml syringe, is inserted into the peritonsillar region in the positions shown in (Figure 13.11). Suction is applied to the syringe and any pus obtained is sent for microbiological examination.

### Incision and drainage

Once again, the area is anaesthetised and the patient prepared. This time an incision is made as shown in Figure 13.11. The incision is opened using sinus forceps and a swab taken for microbiological examination.

When the abscess is decompressed by either of these techniques, the patient gains immediate relief.

# EMERGENCY AIRWAY PROCEDURES

The reader is referred to Chapter 5, pages 57–60.

# HOW TO PERFORM FINE-NEEDLE ASPIRATION CYTOLOGY

The reader is referred to Chapter 8 (page 83).

# 14

# Pharmacology in ENT

Drugs and the ear 164

Drugs and the nose 165

Drugs and the throat 165

There are many drug preparations used in the treatment of ENT disorders. The accessibility of the anatomical areas involved with disease often allows topical agents to be used more than is usual in most other specialities. The information below divides the ENT system up into its constituent parts. The reader will find that similar classes of drugs are used in each area. This is not surprising since they are often affected by similar pathology.

# DRUGS AND THE EAR

## Topical drugs

### Wax removal

- Olive oil and almond oil.
- Sodium bicarbonate is probably more effective as it has been shown not just to soften but to actually dissolve wax.

### Astringents

- Aluminium acetate
- Glycerin and ichthammol

These preparations can be used in otitis externa to reduce meatal swelling by attracting water out of the tissues. Glycerin and ichthammol is very thick and pungent but can occasionally be useful where antibiotic preparations fail.

### Anti-inflammatory/antibiotics

- Steroids, e.g. betamethasone and prednisolone
- Steroid + antibiotic, e.g. hydrocortisone + gentamicin

These preparations are used topically in otitis externa and for infections of the middle ear where there is an abnormal connection to the ear canal, i.e. with a grommet or perforation. They are also used in infections of a surgically created mastoid cavity. The steroid is present to treat the swelling and allergic component of the disease and the antibiotic the infective element. The causative organisms are frequently *Staphylococcus* and *Pseudomonas* and an aminoglycoside will cover both of these. Aminoglycosides are ototoxic in their own right and, if used long term in an ear that has a perforation, may cause labyrinthine damage. However, in short courses, where there is active infection in the middle ear (which is ototoxic as well) and middle-ear mucosal swelling (which helps slow drug absorption into the inner ear), their benefit certainly outweighs any risk.

# Systemic drugs

## Antibiotics

A large number of different organisms are involved in infections of the ear. *Streptococcus pneumoniae* and *Haemophilus influenzae* are often the cause of otitis media, as well as being implicated in infections of the external ear and otitis externa. *Pseudomonas* and sometimes Gram-negative rods are often found in otitis externa. A broad-spectrum penicillin such as amoxycillin, especially when combined with clavulanic acid (Augmentin), is often the drug of choice. Ciprofloxacin is used in more aggressive pseudomonal infections. The exact choice of antibiotic will also depend upon the result of the microbiological culture from the swab. Swabs should always be taken for culture.

## Antiviral agents

Acyclovir can be used in herpes zoster infections which cause the Ramsay Hunt syndrome.

## Vestibular sedatives

- Cinnarizine
- Prochlorperazine

Certain antihistamines and phenothiazines are used for the treatment of vertigo and nausea, resulting from inner and middle-ear conditions. They have a central action which helps relieve the associated nausea and vomiting as well as often having a sedating effect which can be helpful.

## Vasodilator drugs

- Betahistine
- Carbogen

Betahistine is used in the prophylactic treatment of Ménière's disease. Its action seems to be one of vasodilatation and is very useful in some patients. Carbogen is an inhalational agent, a mixture of carbon dioxide and oxygen. It is sometimes used in patients with a sudden-onset sensorineural hearing loss. The high concentration of $CO_2$ causes cerebral dilatation which may improve labyrinthine blood flow and reverse a hearing loss due to a vascular cause.

# DRUGS AND THE NOSE

## Topical drugs

Most topical drugs used in the nose aim to improve nasal airflow and often relieve rhinorrhoea. They work by means of a number of different mechanisms and therefore it is often useful to try an alternative drug type if a patient does not respond to the first preparation.

### Sympathomimetics

- Ephedrine hydrochloride
- Xylometazoline

These sympathomimetics cause vasoconstriction of the nasal mucosa leading to a reduction in its thickness and nasal decongestion. As their effect wears off, rebound vasodilatation occurs and can lead to a worsening, but temporary congestion. Long-term use of these drugs can cause rhinitis medicamentosa and therefore their application should be limited to short courses of 7–10 days.

### Steroids

- Beclomethasone
- Fluticasone

The mainstay of the treatment of rhinitis is topical steroid therapy. Steroids have potent anti-inflammatory effects that reduce mucosal thickness, mucus production and irritation. They are sometimes combined with antibiotics such as neomycin for the treatment of nasal infections.

### Antihistamines

Azelastine hydrochloride modulates the allergic/inflammatory response via the $H_1$-receptors and is used in seasonal allergic rhinitis.

### Antimuscarinics

Muscarinic receptors modulate the secretion from nasal mucosa glands. The muscarinic-receptor blocking agent ipratropium bromide can be effective in helping to treat the watery rhinorrhoea, usually associated with vasomotor rhinitis.

### Mast cell stabilizers

Mast cells play a central role in the inflammatory response of rhinitis and prevention of their activation by sodium cromoglycate can improve nasal symptoms.

## Systemic drugs

### Antibiotics

There are many bacteria that colonize the nose and sinuses and have the ability to cause infection. Streptococci, pneumococci and anaerobic bacteria are commonly involved. A swab should be taken for microbiological culture and this will aid antibiotic choice. Broad-spectrum antibiotics such as amoxycillin are commonly used.

### Antihistamines

- Cetirizine
- Loratadine
- Chlorpheniramine

Systemic antihistamines can be a useful adjunct for the treatment of rhinitis. They can often give good symptomatic relief, especially in 'hayfever' sufferers. The newer drugs are described as non-sedating and can be used regularly.

### Steroids

- Prednisolone
- Dexamethasone

In certain cases, a short course of oral steroids may be warranted in patients with severe symptoms. Gross nasal polyposis, allergic rhinosinusitis and occasionally acute severe rhinitis in schoolchildren around exam time, all can benefit from steroid therapy, often with marked symptomatic control. The risks of oral steroids must, however, be taken into account.

### Decongestants

Pseudoephedrine is a systemic sympathomimetic which is sometimes used as a decongestant preparation. Its use is somewhat limited.

# DRUGS AND THE THROAT

## Topical drugs

### Antiseptics

Oral antiseptics such as chlorhexidine gluconate can be used as gargles or mouthwashes to improve oral hygiene.

## Analgesics

Benzydamine hydrochloride can be useful in oral ulceration, tonsillitis, postsurgery and radiotherapy. Duration of action is often short but can aid systemic analgesia to reduce pain.

## Anti-inflammatory

Corticosteroids, e.g. Adcortyl in Orabase, may be helpful in recurrent aphthous ulceration.

## Antifungal

- Nystatin
- Amphotericin

Fungal infections, such as *Candida albicans*, are a common cause of oral soreness, especially in the debilitated patient. The above drugs are in lozenge or suspension form and are not absorbed systemically.

# Systemic drugs

## Antibiotics

In common with the nose and ear, there are many different organisms that can cause oral and upper aero-digestive tract infections. Streptococci are one of the commonest bacterial causes of tonsillitis and benzylpenicillin is the first line in treatment. Metronidazole seems to be a useful adjunct, but it is best to avoid amoxycillin as this can cause a skin reaction if the infection is actually mononucleosis (glandular fever). Infection due to *Haemophilus influenzae* may now become less common due to the effect of the *Haemophilus influenzae* vaccine.

## Inhalation agents

- Heliox
  This is a mixture of helium and oxygen. Because of the high helium content, this gas is far less dense than air and consequently easier to breathe. Heliox can be used in cases of stridor to improve passage of oxygen through a narrowed larynx and give the surgeon a little extra time to plan any surgical management.
- Carbogen
  This is a mixture of carbon dioxide and oxygen. This causes the blood carbon dioxide level to rise and as a result cerebral perfusion is increased. It is used in cases of sudden-onset sensorineural hearing loss, where a vascular cause is suspected.

# 15

# Glossary of common terms in ENT practice

**Acoustic neuroma**   A slow-growing and benign nerve-sheath tumour of the vestibular nerve (vestibular schwannoma). Usually presents with unilateral sensorineural hearing loss/tinnitus. When large, acoustic neuromas may be life-threatening due to pressure symptoms.

**Anosmia**   Loss of the sense of smell.

**Antrostomy**   A surgically created communication between the maxillary sinus and the nasal cavity. In the past, an artificial hole was created in the inferior meatus. Now, with the advent of functional endoscopic sinus surgery (**FESS**), the antrostomy is made in the middle meatus and is simply an enlargement of the natural sinus ostium.

**Audiogram**   There are two types of audiogram in common practice: A *pure tone audiogram* (PTA) which is a chart showing the hearing thresholds for pure tones against various different frequencies. A *speech audiogram* presents the patient with a series of words at different intensities. The patient is asked to repeat them back to the tester. The number of correct responses is expressed as a percentage for each intensity. This is a test of discrimination.

**Barany box**   This is a clockwork device which is used to create a masking noise when performing Rinne's test.

**BAWO**   Bilateral antral wash-out. The maxillary sinus is cannulated via the inferior meatus. Its contents may be sampled and sent for microbiological examination, and the sinus flushed with sterile water or saline.

**BINA**   Bilateral intranasal antrostomy. See **antrostomy**.

**BINP**   Bilateral intranasal polypectomy.

**'Bo-tox'**   Botulinum toxin. This may be injected into muscles in the treatment of dystonias affecting the larynx, e.g. spasmodic dysphonia, and also in the treatment of torticollis and palatal myoclonus.

**BPPV**   Benign paroxysmal positional vertigo. A common cause of episodic **vertigo**, which occurs when the head is placed in certain conditions. It is believed that the condition is due to displacement of otoliths.

**BSER**   Brainstem evoked response. This is an objective test of hearing. The ear is presented with a series of clicks. With the aid of an averaging computer, the resulting electrical responses which occur in the auditory pathway are recorded.

**Cachosmia**   A sense of an unpleasant smell.

**Caloric tests**   These are tests of labyrinthine function. Cold and warm fluids are flushed into the ear. This causes eddy currents which stimulate the fluid-filled inner ear and nystagmus is induced. Observation and comparison of the responses between the two ears gives an indication of the function of the labyrinth.

**Caldwell–Luc operation**   An operation giving good access to the maxillary sinus via a sublabial approach, in which irreversibly inflamed mucosa is removed. It is less commonly performed since the advent of functional endoscopic sinus surgery (FESS). See **FESS**.

**Choanal atresia**   A congenital failure of development of the posterior part of the nasal passages. The condition may be uni- or bilateral in which case immediate insertion of an oral airway is essential since neonates are obligate nose breathers. The condition may be part of CHARGE, an association of abnormalities which are frequently found in combination (*c*olobomatous malformation; *h*eart defects; *a*tresia of choanae; *r*etardation of growth; *g*enital hypoplasia; *e*ar and oesophageal abnormalities).

**Cholesteatoma**   An epithelial entrapment cyst which most often affects the attic and mastoid. It has the power to erode both bone and soft tissues, and usually presents with an offensive ear discharge.

**Cricothyroidotomy**   A surgically created breathing hole through the cricothyroid membrane.

**CSOM**   Chronic suppurative otitis media.

**Cystic hygroma**   A congenital cavernous lymphangioma commonly affecting the neck and floor of mouth.

**Deltopectoral flap**   An axial pattern, rotation, fasciocutaneous flap, whose blood supply is based on the perforating branches of the internal mammary artery. It may be used in reconstruction of the neck, floor of mouth or oral cavity.

**Dohlman's operation**   An endoscopic operation for pharyngeal pouch. Originally the procedure was performed using diathermy. Nowadays, the technique has been adapted, by the use of a cutting and stapling device to divide the cricopharyngeus muscle which separates the pouch from the lumen of the oesophagus.

**Dysphonia**   An abnormality of voice quality.

**Erythroplakia**   A red patch which occurs on a mucosal surface and from which malignancy can develop.

**FESS**   Functional endoscopic sinus surgery. Here rigid fibreoptic endoscopes are used to perform sinus surgery via the nose. Furthermore, the surgery is concentrated on the middle meatus (**ostiomeatal unit**) where the majority of the sinus ostia open. The concept is that, by performing minimal surgery, in order to restore the natural ventilatory pathways, widespread sinus disease will resolve naturally.

**Free flap**   This describes the movement of a piece of tissue (skin with or without muscle, or with or without bone) with its artery and vein to a distant site where the vessels are connected to local blood supply by microvascular anastomosis. This is required in order to reconstruct a surgically created defect. The most commonly used free flap is the radial free forearm flap.

**Frey's syndrome**   Otherwise known as 'gustatory sweating', this is a rare complication of parotidectomy. Here, the severed postsynaptic secretormotor nerve fibres which normally supply the parotid gland become abnormally redirected and regrow to innervate the sweat glands of the skin. As a result, the patient complains of sweating from the skin overlying the parotid bed during eating.

**Globus syndrome**   This is a sensation of a lump in the throat which is usually intermittent and for which no organic lesion can be found. Previously called 'globus hystericus', this name has been changed to globus syndrome/pharyngeus.

**Glomus tumour**   This is a chemodectoma which arises from glomus bodies of the adventitia of the jugular bulb or along the branches of the tympanic plexus. *Glomus tympanicum* affects the middle ear, *glomus jugulare* affects the internal jugular vein and *glomus vagale* affects the vagus nerve as it leaves the skull base.

**Glottis**   This is the name given to the true vocal cords and the space which lies between them.

**Glue ear**   A collection of fluid, which is often thick and sticky, filling the middle-ear cleft and causing a conductive hearing loss. It is extremely common in childhood and is associated with eustachian tube dysfunction. This condition has several other names: 'secretory or serous otitis media' (SOM), 'otitis media with effusion' (OME) and 'catarrhal otitis'.

**Grommet**   A ventilation or tympanostomy tube which is inserted into the eardrum, used in the treatment of glue ear.

**Inverted papilloma**   Also known as a 'transitional cell papilloma', this is a benign tumour of the nasal cavity which can rarely undergo malignant transformation. It has a tendency to recur unless completely removed. It is named as a result of its infolded histological appearance.

**Keratosis obturans**   An accumulation of debris in the deep ear canal. It may be congenital, in which case it may be associated with bronchiectasis. The acquired form results from a failure of migration of the skin of the deep ear canal, either as a result of radiotherapy or sporadically. The bony ear canal is expanded.

**Laryngectomy**   Surgical removal of the larynx, usually for squamous carcinoma. Most often a total laryngectomy is performed. However, in some circumstances, partial or near total laryngectomy may be preferred.

**Laryngocoele**   This is a hernia of the laryngeal mucosa which arises from the anterior end of the ventricle which in turn lies between the true and false vocal cords. Laryngocoeles may remain confined to the larynx (internal) or may escape to occupy the neck (external).

**Laryngomalacia**   An excessively floppy larynx which may cause stridor in infants and is usually self-limiting.

**Leukoplakia**   This is a white patch which may occur on any mucosal surface and is associated with dysplasia and malignancy.

**Ludwig's angina**   Infection of the submandibular space, usually with haemolytic *Streptococcus*.

**Mastoidectomy**   An operation which removes disease form the mastoid. Various types are employed, the most common being cortical and modified radical.

**Ménière's disease**   A condition believed to be due to abnormal pressures in the fluids of the inner ear (endolymphatic hydrops). The condition presents with episodic attacks of pressure in the ear, tinnitus, hearing loss and vertigo.

**Microlaryngoscopy**   Examination of the larynx using an operating microscope. Delicate microlaryngeal surgery may also be performed using this technique.

**MMA**   Middle meatal antrostomy. See **FESS** and **Antrostomy**.

**Myringitis**   Inflammation of the eardrum.

**Myringoplasty**   An operation to repair a hole in the tympanic membrane.

**Myringotomy**   An incision in the ear drum, most often performed to accommodate grommet insertion.

**Obstructive sleep apnoea**   Apnoea due to upper airways collapse. The chest movements continue in an effort to shift air through the obstructed segment. With time, the blood oxygen saturation levels fall and when critically low levels are reached, a central reflex is activated which causes the patient to waken slightly, and take a deep breath in order to overcome the obstruction. Long term, these periods of desaturation may lead to pulmonary hypertension and right ventricular strain which may lead to ventricular failure, and finally cor pulmonale.

**OME**   Otitis media with effusion. See **Glue ear**.

**Ostiomeatal unit**   The area between the middle turbinate and the lateral wall of the nose into which drain the maxillary, frontal and anterior ethmoidal paranasal sinuses. It is the final common pathway in sinus drainage.

**Otorrhoea**   Ear discharge.

**Otosclerosis**   An abnormal overgrowth of spongy bone in the otic capsule and most importantly around the stapes footplate. Stapes fixation and conductive hearing loss occurs.

**Pectoralis major flap**   The pectoralis major muscle (and overlying skin if necessary) can be mobilized with its blood supply (vascular pedicle) and rotated under a skin tunnel in order to reconstruct a surgically created defect in the neck or oral cavity.

**PGL**   Persistent generalized lymphadenopathy occurs in AIDS patients. It is defined as the presence of symmetrical, mobile and non-tender lymph nodes at least 1 cm in diameter, at two extra-inguinal sites, for three months or more.

**Presbycusis**   The common hearing loss of old age,

caused by the loss of outer hair cells from the cochlea. The pure tone audiogram is diagnostic and shows a symmetrical, high-tone, sensorineural type hearing loss.

**Quinsy**   A paratonsillar abscess.

**Ramsay Hunt syndrome**   This is herpes zoster infection of the geniculate ganglion. It is characterized by facial palsy, vesicles in the ear canal, eardrum and pinna. Also, vertigo and sensorineural hearing loss are occasionally noted.

**Reinke's oedema**   Oedema of the lamina propria of the vocal cords which occurs as a result of smoking.

**Rhinorrhoea**   Nasal discharge.

**Secretory otitis media**   See **Glue ear.**

**Serous otitis media**   See **Glue ear.**

**Sialadenitis**   Inflammation of a salivary gland.

**Sleep apnoea**   This is defined as thirty or more episodes of cessation of breathing each with a minimum duration of 10 seconds, occurring over a 7-hour period of sleep.

**Sleep apnoea index**   This is the number of apnoeic periods per hour.

**SMD**   Submucosal diathermy to the inferior turbinates. Performed to improve nasal air flow in cases of turbinate hypertrophy.

**Snoring**   This is the noise produced in sleep by the vibration of the soft tissues of the pharynx, such as the soft palate and tongue base.

**Stapedectomy**   An operation performed in otosclerosis to restore hearing. It involves removal of the suprastructure of the stapes and its replacement with an artificial piston.

**Stridor**   A high-pitched sound, of musical quality, which occurs as a result of restricted air flow in the upper respiratory tract, usually the larynx.

**Suppurative otitis media**   Suppurative infection of the middle ear and which may be acute or chronic.

**TITs**   Trimming of the inferior turbinates. An operation performed in order to improve nasal air flow.

**T-tube**   A long-term tympanostomy tube (**grommet**) used in patients who suffer from unremitting **glue ear.**

**Tracheostomy**   A surgically created breathing hole in the anterior wall of the trachea.

**Tympanometry**   The indirect measurement of the pressure within the middle ear, or compliance of the eardrum.

**Tympanosclerosis**   White patches on the eardrum which occur as a result of inflammation/trauma to the eardrum. Histologically, these are shown to comprise hyalinized connective tissue. Rarely, tympanosclerosis can affect the middle ear and may cause conductive hearing loss.

**Tympanostomy tube**   See **Grommet.**

**Vertigo**   A sensation of rotary movement.

**Warthin's tumour**   A benign salivary gland tumour, usually arising within the parotid and occasionally bilateral. Also called an 'adenolymphoma'.

# Index

Achalasia, oesophagus 62, 66, 67, 70
Acid reflux, throat 3
Acinic cell, salivary gland 34
Acoustic neuroma 12, 15, 115, 117, 118, 168
Acoustic rhinometry 12, 15
Acoustic trauma 110, 111–12, 118, 119
Acquired immunodeficiency syndrome and HIV 152
  history 3, 4
  neck 81, 83, 86
  oral candidiasis 23
  protection against 153
  salivary gland 34
  sites where infection is manifested 152–3
  sore mouth and oral ulceration 18, 19, 20, 21
  tests and counselling 153
Actinomycosis 34, 86
Acute otitis media 27, 99, 100–1, 106, 117
Acyclovir 19, 117, 164
Adcortyl 166
Adenocarcinoma
  ear 92, 99
  nose 125, 135
  oesophageal 70
  salivary gland 34
  sinus 142
  thyroid 72, 74, 76
Adenoid 26–30, 134
  hypertrophy 102
Adenoid cystic carcinoma 21, 34, 36, 136
Adenoidectomy 27, 102
Adenolymphoma 35
Adenomas
  ear 92, 95, 99
  oesophageal 69
  see also Adenocarcinoma;
    Pleomorphic adenoma
Adenotonsillectomy 29
Adenovirus 23
Agranulocytosis 18, 19
AIDS, see Acquired immunodeficiency syndrome
Air-flow measurements, nasal 15
Air pressure, ear 106
Airway obstruction 64
  children 43, 44–5, 57
Alar cartilage 122
  collapse 10, 123
Alcohol 2, 3
  larynx, disease of 44, 45, 46, 50, 51
  mouth, disease of 21, 22

oesophagus, disease of 70
  snoring and sleep apnoea 28, 29, 30
Allergens 129–30, 133
Allergic rhinitis 16, 125, 129–30, 132
Allergic rhinosinusitis 165
Allergy 2
  nose 126
  testing 15, 16
Almond oil 164
Alport syndrome 110
Aluminium acetate 164
Aminoglycosides 2, 113, 164
Amoxycillin 101, 164, 166
Amphotericin 166
Ampulla 108
Anaemia
  mouth 3, 18
  oesophagus 69, 70
Analgesics 143, 166
Anaplastic carcinoma, thyroid 72, 74
Angiofibroma
  nose and nasopharynx 125, 135, 137
  sinus 142
Angioma 125
Angioneurotic oedema 57
Angiotensin converting enzyme (ACE) 136
Anosmia, see Smell
Antibiotics 143, 164, 165, 166
Anticoagulants 2, 137, 138
Antifungal drugs 166
Antihistamines 130, 133, 164, 165
Anti-inflammatory drugs 164, 166
Antimuscarinics 165
Antinuclear cytoplasmic antibody (ANCA) 136
Antiseptics 165–6
Antispasmodic agents 64
Antitoxin 45
Antiviral agents 164
Antral aspiration, sinus 145
Antro-choanal polyp 133–4
Antrostomy 145, 168, 169
Aphonia 44
Aphthous ulcers 18
Arytenoids 40, 41, 42
Aspergillosis 137
Aspergillus 92, 142, 145
Aspirin
  epistaxis 137
  nasal polyps 125, 132–3, 134
Astringents 164
Atrophic glossitis 69
Atrophic rhinitis 125, 131
Atticotomy 104

Audiogram 5, 119, 168
  cholesteatomas 104
  inner ear 110, 111, 112
  otosclerosis 108
Audiological assessment 119–20
Audiometry 12–14, 16
Auditory nerve 7
Augmentin 164
Aural toilet 91–2, 93, 94, 95, 160–1
Auricle 90–4
  draining a haematoma 161
  examination 5
Auroscope 4, 5, 10
Azelastine hydrochloride 165

Balance 108, 118
Barany noise box 7, 168
Barium swallow 63–4, 65, 66, 67, 68, 70
Barotrauma 99, 106, 142
Basal cell carcinomas
  ear 92, 95
  nose and nasopharynx 123, 125
Basilar membrane 109
Bat ears 91, 92
BAWO (Bilateral antral wash-out) 168
Beclomethasone 165
Behcet's syndrome 18
Bell's palsy 116–17
Benign paroxysmal positional vertigo (BPPV) 110, 114, 117, 120, 168
  bone trauma 112
  Ménière's disease 113
Benign tumour
  ear 99, 106, 117, 169
  larynx 50–1
  mouth 21
  neck 81, 85–6
  nose 134–5
  oesophagus 62, 69
  salivary gland 34, 35–6, 37, 170
  sinus 142
  thyroid 72, 74, 76, 77
Benzydamine hydrochloride 166
Benzylpenicillin 166
Betahistine 113, 114, 164
Betamethasone 164
Betel nut 18, 30
BINA (Bilateral intranasal antrostomy) 168
BINP (Bilateral intranasal polypectomy) 168
Biopsy, neck 84, 87
Bismuth iodide and paraffin paste 157
'Black hairy tongue' 18, 20
Blepharoplasty 138
Blom–Singer valve 50

Blood disorders, mouth 19–20, 21
Bony exostoses, ear 92, 95
'Bo-tox' (Botulinum toxicity) 168
BPPV, see Benign paroxysmal
    positional vertigo
Branchial cyst 81, 84–5, 136
Branchial fistulae 85
Bronchial cancer 53, 55
Brown–Kelly syndrome 62
Brucellosis 86
BSER (Brainstem evoked response) 168
Bulbar palsy 44, 62, 66

Cachosmia 2, 168
Calcification, sinus 145
Calcitonin 74, 75
Caldwell–Luc operation 134, 145, 146,
    168
Caloric tests 168
Cancer, see Malignant tumour
Candida
    AIDS 153
    albicans 166
    ear 92
    mouth 18, 19, 20
    oesophagus 62
    throat 22
Candidiasis, oral 18, 19, 23, 152
Carbimazole 76
Carbogen 164, 166
Carcinoembryonic antigen (CEA) 75
Carcinoma, see Malignant tumour
Carotid aneurysm 81
Carotid artery 32, 80
Carotid body tumours 81
Carotid sheath 32, 81, 82
Cat-scratch fever 86
Cauliflower ear 94, 161
Caustic ingestion 62, 65
Celestin's tube 70
Cerebelo pontine angle (CPA) 114,
    115, 117
Cerebral ischaemia 117
Cerebrospinal fluid 108, 113, 149
    rhinorrhoea 149
Cerebrovascular accident 51, 62, 66
Cerumen, see Wax
Cervical spine 3, 9
Cetirizine 165
Chagas' disease 66
Cheekbone, fracture 148
Chemotherapy, cancer
    larynx 48
    oral cavity 22
Chest X-ray 83
Chickenpox 18
Children, airway 43, 44–5, 57
Chlorpheniramine 165
Choanal atresia 124–5, 168
Cholesteatoma 119, 168
    examination 5, 6
    external ear 92, 95
    history 2, 4
    imaging 14
    inner ear 110, 116, 117, 119
    middle ear 97, 99, 100, 103–6, 118
Chonae 124
Chondromata, larynx 51

Chorda tympani 3, 6, 116
    ear 96, 98
    salivary glands 33, 34
Chordoma 125
Chronic suppurative otitis media
    (CSOM) 99, 100, 102–3, 104,
    118, 119, 168
    aural toilet 160
Cigarette smoking, see Smoking
Ciliary action
    nose 126
    tests 12, 15
    sinuses 140, 141, 142
Cimetidine 65
Cinnarizine 164
Ciprofloxacin 164
Clavicle 9, 80
Cocaine abuse 129
Cochlea 96, 97, 98
    hearing tests 7
    inner ear disorders 111, 113, 119
    mechanism of hearing 109–10
'Coffin corner' 8
Columella 123
    dislocation 123, 128
Computed tomography (CT) 12, 14,
    15–16
    ear 113
    neck 83
    nose 135
    oesophagus 70
    salivary glands 35
    sinus 142–3, 144
    thyroid 76
Congenital abnormalities
    ear 91, 99–100, 110, 118, 119
    oesophagus 62, 63
Continuous positive airway pressure
    ventilation 29
Cooksey–Cawthorne exercises 110, 114
Corticosteroids 166
Counselling, HIV 153
Cranial nerves
    ear 90, 106
    palsy 93
Craniofacial dysostosis 99
Cranio-facial resection 147
Craniopharyngioma 125
Crico-arytenoid muscle 42
Cricoid cartilage 40, 41, 42, 43, 80
Cricopharyngeal myotomy 66, 69
Cricothyroid membrane 80
Cricothyroid muscle 40, 41
Cricothyroidotomy 168
Crocodile forceps 4
Croup 44, 45, 57
Cryptococcus 152, 153
CSOM, see Chronic suppurative otitis
    media
Cystic fibrosis 125, 133
Cystic hygroma 21, 81, 85–6, 168
Cysts, salivary gland 34
Cytology, see Fine-needle aspiration
    cytology
Cytomegalovirus, AIDS 152

De Quervain's thyroiditis 72
Deafness, see Ear

Decongestants 133, 165
Deltopectoral flap 168
Dentures 18
Dermoid
    neck 81, 85, 87
    nose 125
Dew drop nose 131
Dexamethasone 165
Diabetes 20
    mellitus 110
Diathermy 137
Dietary disorders, mouth 19–20, 21
Diphtheria 44, 45
Disseminated intravascular coagulation
    (DIC) 137
Dizziness 2, 120
Dohlman's operation 68, 168
Down's syndrome 99
Drug
    history 2
    ototoxicity 110, 113, 118
    see also Pharmacology
Dynamic video-swallow 66
Dysmorphic nose 125
Dysphagia 67, 68, 69, 70
    investigation 70
    neurological causes 66
Dysphonia 44, 52, 56, 168

EAM, see External auditory meatus
Ear
    AIDS 153
    audiological symptoms, assessment
        119–20
    drugs 164
    examination 5–8
    external ear
        clinical anatomy 90–1
        congenital anomalies 91
        ear wax 91–2
        neoplastic disorders 95
        trauma 93–4
    foreign bodies 158
    hearing loss 118–19
    history 2–3, 4
    inner ear 107–9
        acoustic neuromas and CPA
            tumours 115
        acoustic trauma 111–12
        benign paroxysmal positional
            vertigo 114
        congenital disorders 110
        drug ototoxicity 113
        facial nerve 115–17
        labyrinthitis 110
        mechanism of hearing 109–10
        Ménière's disease 113–14
        presbyacusis 110, 111
        temporal bone trauma 112–13
        tinnitus 118
        vascular disorders 111
        vestibular neuronitis 114
    investigation 12–15
    middle ear
        cholesteatoma 103–6
        clinical anatomy 95–8
        congenital anomalies 99–100
        neoplastic disorders 106

otosclerosis 106–7
symptoms of middle ear disease 99
trauma 106
mop 160–1
syringing 160
tinnitus 118
vertigo 117–18
see also External auditory meatus;
  Otalgia; Otitis externa; Otitis
  media
Eczema 92
Electrical response audiometry 13
Electrocochleography 12, 13
Embolism, ear 111
Emergency airway procedures 57–60
Empyema 64
Encephalitis 62, 66
Encephalocoele, nose 125
Endolymph, ear 108–9
Endoscopy 9, 10
  neck 83
  oesophagus 64, 65, 68, 70
    stapling 68, 69
  sinus 145
Endotracheal intubation 45, 57, 58
Environmental pollutants
  larynx 44, 45, 46, 51
  throat 22
Ephedrine 143, 165
Epiglottis 40, 41, 42
  laryngitis 44
  stridor 57
  tumours 46–7
Epiglottitis 44–5, 57, 152
Epiglottopexy 66
Epilepsy 113
Epistaxis 2, 127, 137, 138
  balloon 157
  stopping 156–7
Epsley's manoeuvre 114
Epstein–Barr virus 136
Equipment 4–5
Erythrocyte sedimentation rate (ESR)
  83, 136, 137
Erythromycin 24, 45
Erythroplakia 20, 21, 30, 168
Ethmoid sinuses 123, 140, 141, 142
  nasal polyposis 132
  sinusitis 144, 145
Eustachian tube 2, 95–8
  barotrauma 106
  middle-ear disease 98–107
  nasopharyngeal carcinoma 125
External auditory meatus (EAM) 90–4,
  96, 97, 98
  examination 5
External laryngocoele 81
Eye trauma, sinus 142

Facial cellulitis 92
Facial fracture 142, 148–9
Facial nerve 115–17
  cholesteatoma 104
  ear 93, 97, 98, 99
  history 3
  palsy
    ear 103, 104, 105, 112, 116, 117
    salivary glands 34, 36

salivary glands 32, 33, 34, 36
stapedial reflex 14
Facial pain 2
Facial plastic surgery 137–8
Facial trauma 142, 148–9
Facial weakness 3
Fallopian canal 97
Fenestration 60
FESS (Functional endoscopic sinus
  surgery) 145, 168
Fibreoptic endoscope 9, 10
Fibroma
  larynx 51
  nose 125
Fibrous dysplasia, sinus 142
Fine-needle aspiration (FNA) 35
Fine-needle aspiration cytology
  (FNAC)
  neck 83, 85, 86, 87
  thyroid 76
Fistula test 104
Fluroscopy 66, 70
Fluticasone 165
Folate 18, 19
Foley urinary catheter 157
Follicular adenocarcinoma, thyroid 72,
  74, 76
Follicular tonsillitis 23
Foreign bodies
  ear 92, 94, 106, 118
  larynx 57
  nose 125, 127–8
  oesophagus 62–4
  removal 157–60
Fracture
  facial 142, 148–9
  nose 125, 126, 127
Free field test 7–8
Free flaps 22, 168
Free jejunal grafting 69, 70
Frey's syndrome 37, 168–9
Frontal sinus 140, 141, 145–6
Fronto-ethmoidectomy 146
Frusemide 113
Full blood count (FBC) 83
Functional dysphonia 44, 52, 56
'Functional endoscopic sinus surgery'
  (FESS) 145, 168
Fungal infection
  AIDS 152
  ear 93
  larynx 45
  sinusitis 145
Furuncle
  ear 92
  neck 81

Gastro-oesophageal reflex 22, 46
  disease (GORD) 62, 64–5
Gastrostomy 66, 70
Gene markers 48
Gentamicin 113, 164
Glandular fever
  drugs 166
  neck 81, 83, 86
  nose 136
  sore throat and tonsillitis 22, 23, 24,
    25

Glioma, nose 125
Globus pharyngeus 65
Globus syndrome 169
Glomus tumours 99, 106, 117, 169
Glossopharyngeal nerve 33
Glossitis 69
Glottis 169
  see also Vocal cord/fold
Glucose test 149
Glue ear 99, 100, 101–2, 104, 106, 119
  adenoid 27
  AIDS 153
  nasopharynx 136
  rhinitis 129
Glycerin 164
Goitre 72, 73, 74, 76, 81
GORD (Gastro-oesophageal reflux
  disease) 62, 64–5
Gouty tophi 92
Granulomatous disease
  ear 119
  nose 136–7
  salivary gland 34, 35
Graves' disease 72, 73, 75
Greater auricular nerve 90
Grommet 169
  cholesteatoma 104
  ear wax 92
  Meniere's disease 114
  otitis media 101–2, 106
Gustatory sweating 37

H$_2$–receptor antagonist 65
Haemangiomas
  larynx 44, 51
  mouth 21
  salivary gland 34
Haematoma
  auris 94, 161
  pinna 161
  salivary glands 37
Haemophilia 137
Haemophilus 142
  influenzae 23, 45, 101, 164, 166
Hairy leukoplakia 19, 20, 152
Hallpike manoeuvre 114
Hashimoto's thyroiditis 72, 75
Hayfever 2, 126, 130, 165
Head mirror 4–5
Head trauma
  ear 106, 113, 117, 119
  sinus 142
Hearing
  mechanism of 109–10
  see also Ear; Otology
Hearing aid 100, 102, 108 ,110
Hearing tests, see Otology
Heartburn 64
Heliox 166
Hemilaryngectomy 48
Hereditary haemorrhagic telangiectasia
  (HHT) 137
Hernia
  hiatus 62, 64–5
  neck 87
Herpes 92
  simplex 18–19, 23, 152
  zoster 19, 117, 164

Hilar lymph nodes 62
Histamine 130
*Histoplasmas* 153
History 2–4
    ear 2–3
    mouth and neck 3–4
    nose 2, 4
    structure of 2
    throat 3
HIV, *see* Acquired immunodeficiency
    syndrome and HIV
Hoarseness, voice 4, 9, 44, 51–6
Honeymoon rhinitis 131
Hormonal manipulation, thyroid 76
Human immunodeficiency virus, *see*
    Acquired immunodeficiency
    syndrome and HIV
Human papilloma virus (HPV) 51
Hurtle cell tumour, thyroid 72
Hydrocortisone 164
Hyoid bone 80
Hyperkeratosis 20
Hypernasality 27
Hypersensitivity reaction Type 1
    129–30
Hypertension, epistaxis 137, 138
Hyperthyroidism 75, 76
Hypocalcaemia 73, 77
Hypoglossal nerve 32, 33, 34
Hypoplasia, sinus 142
Hypothyroidism 73, 75, 76
Hysterical dysphonia 44, 56

Ichthammol 164
Imaging
    otology 12, 14–15
    rhinology 15–16
Impedance audiometry 12, 14, 16, 170
Impetigo 92
Immunoglobulins 16, 129–30
Incus 6, 95, 96, 98, 107
Infections, neck 86
Infectious mononucleosis, *see*
    Glandular fever
Infective lymphadenopathy 86
Infective pharyngitis 22–3
Infective rhinitis 129, 132
Infective ulcers of the mouth 18–19
Inferior constrictor muscle 67
Influenza 23
Inhalation agents 166
Intrauterine infection 110
Inverted papilloma 169
    nose 125, 135
    sinus 142
Iodine deficiency, goitre 73
Ipratropium bromide 130, 165
Iron deficiency 18, 19, 69

Jacobson's nerve 33
Jobson horn probe 4, 158, 160
Jugulodigastric lymph node 80, 81
Juvenile angiofibroma 135, 137

Kaposi's sarcoma 19, 152, 153
Keratoconjunctivitis sicca 35
Keratosis obturans 92, 118, 169
Killian's dehiscence 67, 87

*Klebsiella* 137
Koilonychia 69

Labyrinth 107–17
Labyrinthectomy 114
Labyrinthine concussion 110, 112
Labyrinthitis 105, 110, 113, 114, 117,
    118, 119, 120
Lacrimal gland 34
Larygocoele 44
Laryngeal
    cleft 44
    diphtheria 44, 45
    muscles 41–2, 43
    neoplasia 46–51, 65
    nerve 52–3, 72, 73, 77, 90
        palsy 44, 52–3
    web 44
Laryngectomy 48–50, 51, 66, 70, 169
Laryngitis
    acute 44–5
    chronic 45–6, 65
Laryngocoele 81, 87, 169
Laryngomalacia 44, 57, 169
Laryngoscopy 9, 53
Laryngotomy 58
Laryngotracheobronchitis, acute 45
Larynx, diseases of 43–4
    AIDS 152
    emergency airway procedures 57–60
    examination 9
    hoarseness 51–6
    infective and inflammatory
        conditions 44–6
    neoplasms 4, 44, 46–51, 65
    stridor 56–7
    structure and function 40–3
Laser palatal scarring 29–30
Lateral cartilage, nose 122
Lateral rhinotomy 147
Le Fort fractures 148
Leiomyoma 69
Leprosy 45
Lethal midline granuloma 136
Leukaemia 18, 19, 137
Leukoplakia 18, 20, 21, 30, 169
    hairy 19, 20, 152
Lichen planus 18, 20
Light reflex 5, 6, 96
Lingual nerve 32, 33, 34
Lipoma
    neck 81
    oesophageal 69
    salivary gland 34
Little's area 123, 124, 138
Loratadine 165
Lower motor neurone, facial nerve
    116
Ludwig's angina 86, 169
Lymphadenitis 81
Lymphangioma 85–6
Lymphoepithelioma 136
Lymphomas
    AIDS 152, 153
    neck 4, 83, 84, 87, 136
    nose 136
    throat 22
    thyroid 72

Macula 108
Magnetic resonance imaging (MRI) 12,
    15, 16
    ear 115, 118
    neck 83
    oesophagus 70
    thyroid 76
Malignant tumour 2, 4
    AIDS 152–3
    ear 92, 93, 94, 95, 99, 106, 115,
        117
    larynx 43, 44, 46–50, 53, 55, 57
    mouth 18, 19, 21–2, 24, 30
    neck 81, 83, 86–7
    nose 123, 125, 134, 135–6, 137
    oesophagus 62, 65, 68, 70
    pharynx 90
    salivary gland 21, 34, 36, 37
    sinus 142, 147–8
    thyroid 72, 73–4, 76, 77, 81
Malleus 95, 96, 97, 98
    examination 5, 6
Mast cell stabilizers 165
Mastoid 80, 95, 96, 97, 98
    examination 9
Mastoidectomy 104, 105, 169
Mastoiditis 105
Maxillary fractures 148
Maxillary sinus 123, 140, 141
Maxillectomy 147, 148
Measles 18
Meatus 118, 124
    stenosis 93
Mediastinitis 64, 65
Medullary carcinoma, thyroid 72, 74
Melanoma 92
Ménière's disease 110, 113–14, 119,
    169
    drugs 164
    tinnitus 118
    vertigo 117, 120
Meningioma 99
Meningitis 2, 115, 119, 149, 153
Meningocoele, nose 125
Mentoplasty 138
Metronidazole 166
Micrognathia 30
Microlaryngoscopy 51, 169
MMA (Middle meatal antrostomy)
    145, 168, 169
Modiolus 109
Monospot test
    neck lumps 83
    tonsillitis 24
Motor neurone disease 44, 52, 62, 66
Mouth
    AIDS 152
    examination 8–9
    history 3–4
    lumps and swellings 21–2
    sore mouth and oral ulceration
        18–21
MRI scan, *see* Magnetic resonance
    imaging
Mucocoeles 144
Mucocutaneous junction 123
Muco-epidermoid tumours 34, 36
Mucoperichondrium 123

Mucoperiostium 123–4
Mucosa 10
Mucosal wave 41, 42
Mucus retention cysts 21
Mueller manoeuvre 29
Multiple endocrine neoplasia syndrome 74
Multiple sclerosis
  ear 113, 115, 117, 119, 120
  larynx 51
  oesophagus 62, 66
Mumps 34, 110
Myasthenia gravis 62, 66
*Mycoplasmal infection* 133
Myocutaneous flap reconstruction 69, 70
Myringitis 169
Myringoplasty 103, 169
Myringotomy 106, 169

Nasal
  adhesions 131, 132
  agenesis 125
  cavity 140, 141
  polyposis 125, 132–4, 135, 142, 147
    drugs 165
  septum 123, 124
    choanal atresia 129
    deviation 128
    haematoma 126, 127, 129
    perforation 129
    surgery 128–9
  tampons 157
  valve 123
  vestibule 122–3
  see also Nose
Naso-endoscopy, sleep 29, 30
Nasogastric tube 66
Nasolacrimal duct 124
Nasopharynx, see Nose
Nausea 64, 164
Neck
  clinical anatomy 80–2
  congenital neck remnants 84–6
  examination 9
  hernias 87
  history 3–4
  infections 86
  investigation of neck lumps 3–4, 82–4
  lymph node enlargement 86–7
  nodes 153
Neomycin 165
Neonatal trauma 2
Neoplasia
  ear 92, 95, 99, 106, 118, 119
  larynx 4, 44, 46–51, 65
  neck 3–4, 86
  salivary glands 34, 35–6
  throat 3
  thyroid 73–4, 77
Neoplastic lymphadenopathy 86
Neurodermatitis 92
Neuroepithelium 108, 109
Neurogenic tumour 99
Neurology
  dysphagia 66
  hoarseness 52–5
  see also Facial nerve

Neuroma
  acoustic 12, 15, 115, 117, 118, 168
  vagal 62, 66, 81
Neuronitis, vestibular 114, 117
Noise, acoustic trauma 110, 111–12, 118, 119
Non-granulomatous infection 136–7
Non-Hodgkin's lymphoma 152
Non-steroidal anti-inflammatory drugs 137, 138
Nose and nasopharynx
  AIDS 152, 153
  blocked and runny nose 126–32
  drugs 165
  epitaxis 137
  eustachian tube 98
  examination 10
  foreign bodies 158–9
    fracture nose 126
  granulomatous and non granulomatous injection 136–7
  growths, tumours and destructive lesions 2, 4, 125, 134–6
  history 2, 4
  investigation 15–16
  nasal polyposis 132–4, 142, 147, 165
  olfaction tests 12, 15
  rhinology 15–16
  rhinoplasty and facial plastic surgery 137–8
  structure and function 122–5
Nose bleed, see Epistaxis
Nystagmus 104, 113, 114
Nystatin 166

Obstructive sleep apnoea 169
  syndrome (OSAS) 24, 25, 26, 27–30, 102
Obturator 147, 148
Oesophagus
  achalasia 66
  caustic ingestion 65
  congenital abnormalities 62
  dysphagia
    investigation 70
    neurological causes 66
  foreign bodies 62–4
  gastro-oesophageal reflux disease and hiatus hernia 64–5
  pharyngeal pouch 66–9
  postcricoid web 69
  speech 49
  structure and function 62
  tumours 4, 62, 69–70
Olfaction, see Smell
Olfactory neuroblastoma 125
Olive oil 164
OME (Otitis media with effusion), see Glue ear
Omeprazole 65
Oncocytoma
  nose 125
  salivary gland 34
Oral candidiasis 18, 19, 23, 152
Oral cavity, see Mouth

Orbit 123
  blow-out fracture 149
Organ of Corti 109
Oropharynx 3, 4
Osseous spiral lamina 109
Ossicles 14, 95–107, 109, 118
  adhesions 101
  dislocation 99
  examination 6, 7
Osteitis 93
Osteoma 99, 125, 142
Osteomeatal unit 140, 141, 169
Osteomyelitis 93, 95
Otalgia 90, 91, 99
  history 2, 3
  oral cavity cancers 22
  tonsillitis 25
Otitis externa 91, 92–3, 94, 95
  AIDS 153
  aural toilet 160
  drugs 164
Otitis media 98, 99, 100
  acute 27, 99, 100–1, 106, 117, 118, 119
  AIDS 153
  inner ear 110
  see also Chronic suppurative otitis media
Otitis media with effusion (OME), see Glue ear
Otoacoustic emissions 12, 13–14
Otoliths 108, 112, 114
Otology, investigations 12
  auroscope 5
  electrical response audiometry 13
  imaging 14–15
  impedance audiometry 14
  otoacoustic emissions 12, 13–14
  pure tone audiogram 12
  simple tests 7–8
  speech audiogram 12–13
  stapedial reflexes 12, 14, 108
  tuning fork tests 5–7, 12, 99, 104, 108
Otorrhoea 169
  history 2, 4
  inner ear 113
  middle ear 99, 100, 103, 104, 106
  otitis externa 92
Otosclerosis 99, 106–7, 108, 110, 118, 119, 169
Oval window 98, 99, 108, 109, 110, 118
  rupture 113

Pan-endoscopy 21, 30, 50, 70, 83
Papillary adenocarcinoma, thyroid 72, 74
Papilloma
  ear 92, 95
  larynx 44, 50–1, 57
  nose 123, 125, 134–5, 137
  see also Inverted papilloma
Paracetamol 143
Paracusis willsii 107
Parainfluenza 23
Paramyxovirus 34

Paranasal sinuses 122, 124, 125, 140
  AIDS 152
  facial trauma 148–9
  history 2, 3
  sinusitis 142–7
  structure and function 140–2
  tumours 147–8
  *see also* Sinusitis
Para-oesophageal abscess 64
Parapharyngeal abscess 86
Parapharyngeal space, neck 82
Parathyroid glands 77
Parotid gland 32–7, 80
  AIDS 153
  examination 9
Parotidectomy 95
Pars flaccida 96, 97, 98
Pars tensa 96, 97
Patterson operation 146
Patterson syndrome 62
Paul Bunnell test 24, 83
Peak inspiratory nasal air flow 12, 15
Pectoralis major flap 169
Pellagra 19
Pemphigus, autoimmune 18
Penicillin 24, 45, 164
Perforation, ear 92, 99, 100, 102–3,
  113, 119
Perichondritis 92, 93
Perilymph 108, 109
Perinatal hypoxia 110
Periorbital cellulitis 143, 144, 147
Peritonsillar abscess, *see* Quinsy
Pernicious anaemia 69
Persistent generalized
  lymphadenopathy (PGL) 153, 169
Petrositis 105
PGL (Persistent generalized
  lymphadenopathy) 153, 169
Pharmacology 164
  ear 164
  nose 165
  throat 165–6
Pharyngeal pouch 62, 66–9, 81, 87
Pharyngitis 22–3
Phenothiazines 164
Pierre–Robin syndrome 99
Pinna, *see* Auricle
Pinnaplasty 138
Plasmacytoma 125
Plastic surgery 137–8
Pleomorphic adenoma
  mouth 21
  salivary glands 34, 35, 36, 37
*Pneumococcus* 23, 165
*Pneumocystis* 153
  *carinii* 153
Poisons 65
Polio 66
Polyarteritis nodosa 110
Polycythaemia 18, 19
Polypectomy 133, 168
Polyps, *see* Nasal polyposis
'Pope otowicks' 161
Post Nasal Space (PNS) 124–5, 134
Postcricoid web 62, 69
Pre-auricular sinuses 91
Prednisolone 164, 165

Pregnancy
  goitre 72, 73
  rhinitis 131
Presbyacusis 110, 111, 117, 118, 119,
  169–70
Pretracheal fascia 81, 82
Prochlorperazine 164
Proof puncture, sinus 145
Propylthiouracil 76
Pseudoephedrine 165
*Pseudomonas* 92, 93, 103, 164
Pseudosalivary swellings 36
Psoriasis 92
Pulsus paradoxicus 58
Pure tone audiogram 12, 16
Pyriform fossa 4, 41, 42, 90
Pyriform sinus 41

Quinsy 22, 24, 25, 170
  draining 161–2

Radioactive ablation, thyroid 76, 77
Radio-Allergo-Absorbent Test (RAST)
  12, 16
Radioisotope scanning, thyroid 76
Radiotherapy
  laryngeal cancer 48, 49
  sinuses 147–8
Ramsay Hunt syndrome 116, 117,
  164, 170
Ranitidine 65
Ranula 21
Rapid eye movement (REM) 29
'Reactionary haemorrhage' 25, 27
Reactive lymphadenitis 81
Recurrent laryngeal nerve palsy 44,
  52–3
Reinke's oedema 44, 45, 46, 55, 170
Reissner's membrane 109, 113
Retraction pocket, cholesteatoma 103
Retrocochlea, pathology 114, 119
Retromandibular vein 32
Retropharyngeal space 82
Rhabdomyosarcoma 125
Rhesus incompatibility 110
Rhinitis 125, 129, 131, 165
  allergic rhinitis 16, 125, 129–30, 132
  atrophic rhinitis 125, 131
  medicamentosa 130–1, 165
  sicca 131
  simple acute infective rhinitis 129
  vasomotor rhinitis 125, 130, 165
Rhinolalia-aperta 27
Rhinolith 127
Rhinology, *see* Nose and nasopharynx
Rhinophyma 122, 125
Rhinoplasty 137–8
Rhinorrhoea 126, 170
  adenoidal conditions 26
  AIDS 152
  drugs 165
  facial trauma 149
  history 2, 4
  nasal polyposis 134
  rhinitis 129, 130, 132
  tumours 137
Rhinosinusitis 22, 142, 145
  allergic 165

Rhinosporidiosis 137
Rhinovirus 23
Rinnes test 7, 8, 12, 99, 108, 118
Romberg's test 118
Round window 96, 98, 99, 108, 110
  examination 6
  hearing 109
  rupture 113
Rubella 110

Saccharin taste test 12, 15
Saccule 107, 108, 109, 114
Salivary glands
  AIDS 153
  diseases 34–6
  fistula 37
  history 3
  innervation 33–4
  nucleus 33, 34
  structure and function 32
  surgery 36–7
  tumours 21
Sarcoidosis 18, 34, 125, 129, 136–7
Sarcoma
  Kaposi's 19, 152, 153
  sinus 142
Scala media 109
Scala vestibuli 109
Scala tympani 109
Scarlet fever 18
Scleroderma 62
Scleroma 45, 125, 129, 137
Screamer nodules 44, 52, 55, 56
Scurvy 19
Seasonal allergic rhinitis 165
Sebaceous cysts, neck 81
Secondary haemorrhage 25, 27
Secretory otitis media (SOM), *see* Glue
  ear
Semicircular canals 107–8, 109
Senile rhinitis 131
Septoplasty 128
Septum 10
Serous otitis media, *see* Glue ear
Sialadenitis 34, 35, 37, 81, 82, 170
Sialography 35
Sialolithiasis 34, 35, 37
Sickle cell disease 129
Silolithiasis 81, 82
Silver Nitrate cautery stick 4
Singer's nodules 44, 52, 55, 56
Sinus, *see* Paranasal sinuses
Sinus ostia 142, 143
Sinusitis 140, 142
  acute 142–4, 147
    acute frontal 143–4, 147
    mucocoeles 144
    periorbital cellulitis 144
  chronic 142, 145–7
    fungal 145
  *see also* Rhinosinusitis
Sjogren's syndrome 34, 35
Skin tests 12, 16
Sleep apnoea 26, 27–30, 170
  central 28
  index 28, 170
  obstructive 28
Sleep nasendoscopy 29, 30

SMD (Submucosal diathermy) 131, 170
Smell 122
  loss of 2, 168
  tests for 12, 15
Smoking
  history 2, 3
  larynx 44, 45, 46, 49, 51, 56
  mouth 21, 22, 30
  oesophagus 70
Sneezing 2
Snoring 26, 27–30, 56–7, 170
Social history 2
Sodium bicarbonate 164
Sodium cromoglycate 130, 165
Sore throat 3, 22–6
Speech audiogram 12–13
Sphenoid sinus 140, 141, 142
Spice, chewing 18, 30
Squamous cell carcinoma
  ear 92, 94, 95, 99, 106, 117
  larynx 44, 46–50, 51
  mouth 19, 21–2, 30
  neck 86–7
  nose 123, 125, 134, 135, 137
  oesophageal 70
  sinus 142
  throat 22
Stapedectomy 5, 107, 108, 170
Stapes 95, 96, 98, 107, 109
  examination 6
  reflexes 12, 14, 108
*Staphylococcus* 92, 164
Stenosis
  meatal 93
  oesophagus 62, 63
  subglottic 44, 57
  vestibular 125
Sternomastoid muscle 9, 80, 82
Steroids 164, 165
  Bell's palsy 116
  granulomatous infection 136
  nasal polyposis 133, 134
  rhinitis 130, 131, 132, 136
'Stertor' 56–7
Stewart's granuloma 136
Stomach pull-up 69, 70
Stomatitis 69
Strawberry tongue 18
*Streptococcus* 23, 142, 164, 165, 166
  *pneumoniae* 101
  *viridans* 86
Streptomycin 137
Stridor 45, 51, 56–7, 170
Stroboscope 41
Stylomastoid foramen 98
Subglottis 41, 43, 46–7
  stenosis 44, 57
Sublingual gland 32–7
Submandibular duct 32, 33
Submandibular gland 9, 32–7, 80
Submandibular space 82
Submucus diathermy (SMD) 131, 170
Submucus resection 128
Suppurative otitis media 170
  *see also* Chronic suppurative otitis media
Supraglottis 41, 42–3, 44, 46–7, 152

Swallowing 40–1
  *see also* Dysphagia
Sympathomimetics 165
Syphilis 18, 19
  ear 113
  larynx 44, 45
  nose 125, 129, 137
  throat 23
Syringing, ear 91–2, 160

Tabes dorsalis 66
Taste 3
T-cell lymphoma
  nose and nasopharynx 125, 136
  sinus 142
Tectorial membrane 109
Teeth 3
Temporal bone trauma 99, 110, 112–13
Temporomandibular joint 3
Thermal trauma 92, 94
Thiouracil 34
Throat
  drugs 165–6
  foreign bodies 159–60
  history 3, 4
  sore throat and tonsillitis 22–6
Thudicums nasal speculum 4, 10, 157
Thyroglobulin 75
Thyroglossal cyst 72, 81, 84
Thyroglossal fistula, neck 84
Thyroid gland 80, 82, 87
  autoantibodies 75
  cartilage 40, 41, 42, 43
  clinical anatomy 72
  ear 110
  enlargement 62
  examination 9, 83
  function tests 75
  goitre 73
  history 4
  investigation of thyroid disease 75–6
  neoplastic conditions 73–4, 81
  treatment of thyroid conditions 76–7
Thyroid-stimulating hormone (TSH) 73, 75, 76
Thyroidectomy 73, 74, 75, 76–7
Thyroiditis 72, 75, 81
Thyroplasty 54
Thyrotoxicosis 74
Thyroxine (T4) 74, 75, 76
Tinnitus 118
  external ear 91
  history 2
  inner ear 108, 110
    acoustic trauma 111–12
    benign paroxysmal positional vertigo 114
    facial nerve 115, 117
    Ménière's disease 113
  middle ear 99, 106, 107
TITs (Trimming of the inferior turbinates) 170
TNM classification, malignancy 47–8, 86
Tongue 8, 30
  'black hairy tongue' 18, 20
  malignancy 4

Tonsils 4, 9
Tonsillectomy 24–6, 29, 102
Tonsillitis 3, 19, 22, 23–6, 166
Topical drugs 165
Torus palitinus 21
Toxoplasmosis 81, 83, 86
Trachea 80
Tracheo-oesophageal fistula 49, 62, 63, 64
Tracheostomy 58–60, 170
  dysphagia 66
  hoarseness 55
  inflammation larynx 45
  neoplasms 51
  snoring and sleep apnoea 30
β-Transferrin 149
Transitional cell papilloma, nose 135
Trauma
  ear 92, 93–4, 106, 110, 111–12, 119, 120
  facial 142, 148–9
  facial nerve 117
  larynx 44, 57
  middle ear 106
  mouth 18, 21
  nose 126, 127, 128, 129
  ulcers 18
Treacher Collins syndrome 91
Trench mouth 19
Trephination 145–6
Trigeminal nerve 33, 90
Tri-iodothyronine (T3) 75
Trismus 24
T-tube (Long-term tympanostomy tube) 170
Tuberculosis
  larynx disease 44, 45
  neck disease 81, 86
  nose disease 125, 129, 136, 137
  salivary glands disease 34, 35
  sinus disease 142
  throat disease 23
Tuberculous otitis media 99
Tumours
  ear 2, 113
  nose 2, 129
  oesophageal 66
  sinuses 147–8
  *see also* Benign tumour; Malignant tumour
Tuning fork tests 5–7, 12, 99, 104, 108
Turbinates 123–4
  examination 10
  rhinitis 130–1
  sinuses 140, 141
  surgery 131–2
Turbinectomy 131–2
Tympanic membrane 90, 92, 95–107, 109, 118, 119
  acoustic trauma 111
  otitis externa 93
  temporal bone trauma 113
Tympanic plexus 33
Tympanometry 12, 14, 16, 170
Tympanosclerosis 101, 103, 170
Tympanostomy tube, *see* Grommet

Ultrasound scan
  neck 83
  thyroid 76
Upper motor neurone, facial nerve 116
Utricle 107, 108, 109
Uvulopharyngopalatoplasty (UPPP) 24, 29

Vagal neuroma 62, 66, 81
Vagal stimulation 90
Vascular disorders, ear 110, 111, 118, 119, 120
Vasculitis 110
Vasodilator drugs 164
Vasomotor rhinitis 125, 130, 165
Vertigo 117–18, 120, 170
  benign paroxysmal positional vertigo 110, 112, 113, 114, 117, 168
  drugs 164
  labrynthitis 110
  Ménière's disease 113
  temporal bone trauma 112
  trauma, middle ear 106
Vestibular neuronitis 114, 117, 120
Vestibular sedatives 164

Vestibular system 107–17, 125
Vestibulitis 125, 127
Vibrissae 122
Vincent's organism 19
Viral pharyngitis 22–3
Viral warts 134–5
Vitamin $B_{12}$ 18, 19
Vitamin C 18, 19
Vocal cord/fold 41, 42–57
  check, thyroid surgery 77
  fixation 44
  medialization 54–5, 66
  nodules 55
  palsy 9, 44, 53–5, 57
  polyps and cysts 44, 52, 55–6, 57
  web 57
Vocal polyp 44, 52, 57
Vocal tract 40
Voice 3
  hoarseness 4, 9, 44
  restoration, laryngeal cancer 49–50
Von Willebrand's disease 137

Waardenburg syndrome 110
Warfarin 137

Warthin's tumour 34, 35, 36, 170
Waterbrash 64
Wax 2, 90, 91–2, 95, 118
  drugs 164
Weber's test 7, 12, 99, 108, 118
Weber–Fergusson incision 147
Wegener's granulomatosis
  ear 99, 110, 111
  mouth 18
  nose 125, 129, 136
Wharton's duct 9, 32–7, 80
Whisper test 7–8
White cell count 83

Xerostomia 35
X-ray 15
  neck lumps 83
  oesophagus 63–4
  sinus 142–3
Xylometazoline 165

Young's operation 137

Zoster virus 23
Zygoma, fractures 148, 149